101 NIGHTS OF GREAT SEX™

BY

LAURA CORN

PARK AVENUE PUBLISHERS

PUBLISHED BY PARK AVENUE PUBLISHERS, INC.

Los Angeles, California

Send all inquiries to: parkavenuepublishers@gmail.com (310) 392-0641

ISBN: 978-0-578-55166-1

www.101Nights.com

www.LauraCorn.com

Second Print Run of 2020 edition

DISCLAIMER Please read before proceeding

This book is sold with the understanding that it is intended solely for the use of informed, consenting, and hopefully monogamous adults who want to rejuvenate, enliven, and sustain a great sexual relationship. The author is not a medical doctor or therapist; she has, however, intensely studied this subject for the past past 25 years and is the best-selling author of 9 books in this genre. Almost every recipe in this book has been recommended by leading sexual therapists.

WARNING: The reader is cautioned that following the suggestions and scenarios herein is strictly voluntary and at the reader's own risk and discretion. Also, this book contains suggestions of sex acts that are illegal in some states. Know your state's laws about sex and break them at your own risk. The positions and products mentioned in this book are safe and satisfying for the majority of adult women and men. Every individual is unique; therefore, you should not employ any position, technique or product that is not suitable to your physical or sexual limitations.

The author, publisher, and distributor do not endorse any specific product or assume any product liability for any product mentioned in the book. The choices and responsibility for any consequences which may result from the use of any product or following any suggestion or scenario herein belong to the reader.

The author and Park Avenue Publishers, Inc., Los Angeles, shall have neither liability nor responsibility to any person or entity with regard to any losses or damage caused or alleged to be caused, either directly or indirectly, by the information contained in this book.

Book Design by Doris Jew
Icons Designed by Paul Payongayong (paulpayongayong.tumblr.com)

ACKNOWLEDGEMENTS

This book is dedicated with deepest love and affection to my lover and partner, Jeff Petersen. Without you there would be no Great Sex, either in print or in my life.

I am also deeply indebted to a host of people who made this book possible. I have been especially fortunate to have so many wonderful teachers, friends and business associates. To each of them, I extend my heartfelt gratitude:

Marty Bishop, DJ extraordinaire, whose fertile imagination and flair permeate this book.

Leo Damian, my dear friend. There would be no 2020 edition without your contribution. I love you!

Anna del Gaizo, my amazing editor. There's no way I could have pulled off this amount of great sex without your skills.

Stephanie Teobold, my brilliant contributor. Your drive to explore and push boundaries (sex and otherwise!) has inspired me endlessly.

Charlie Ilgunas, my copyeditor, whose hard work, exuberance, and eagle eye have been invaluable. I wish him a bright future as an editor!

Alan Rommelfanger the best PR guy in the world!!!!

Rachel May Stafford, Tina Macintosh, Joe Ullrich, Amanda Barnett, and Rich Lippman for exercising their writing chops on seduction titles. Chow Down, Baby!

Stacie Anthony, my wonderful assistant for the past 7 years.

Rodrigo Corral, incredible graphic designer, who took this book and made it a work of art. A gazillion thanks for bringing your remarkable talent to this project. I would also like to thank Rodrigo's assistant, Rachel Adam, who kept everything on track.

Doris Jew, for her work implementing the entire book's design. It's always a joy working with you, Doris. You are one of the hardest working, most skillful designers on planet Earth.

Nikki Groom, trailblazing ink slinger & digital scribe.

Jen Bergstrom and Simon & Schuster for allowing me to print seductions from the best-selling book, *Passport To Pleasure*.

Paul Joannides, Dr. Sadie Allison, Chip Rowe, Tracy Cox, Leslie Swartz, Tim Daze, Andrea Skelton, Nicky Curranza, Robin Eisenman, the entire staff at the Doves Beauty Salon in Santa Monica, and the sexy B-school Babes.

I'd also like to thank all the people who bought my books, responded to me on the air, stood in line for hours for a personal word with me, endured my probing interviews and opened up their hearts, minds, and souls to provide me with the most essential ingredient in this book: their desires, needs and experiences. Without you, this book truly would not be possible.

TABLE OF CONTENTS

INTRODUCTION TO GREAT SEX

Is YOUR SEX LIFE PERFECT?

Are you totally thrilled, aroused, and satisfied after every erotic encounter? Is your life behind the bedroom door absolutely, completely, overwhelmingly fulfilling?

Then put this book down!!

Somebody else needs it more than you.

Most of us, in fact, find it all too easy to let *life* get in the way of love. Jobs and bills and chores and kids all conspire to push intimacy to the bottom of our list of priorities. If we can make any private time at all for each other, it's only when we're tired and distracted. The same old moves, the same old positions, and after a while sex gets, well—

Boring. Boooorr-ing.

In survey after survey, boring sex is the number-one complaint of couples across the country. In fact, in 2019, while sex positivity is seemingly at an all-time high, people are statistically having less sex than ever. And it doesn't have to be that way.

Because this book guarantees great sex. 101 Nights of it, just like the title says.

That's every week, twice a week, for one full year. Now, I know that's a lot to ask from one little book! But I promise you that it works. Here's how—

Every week, you and your partner flip through the titles, discussing the ones that catch your eye. This can be a real blast—it's a little like window-shopping for sex. Each of you then tears a page from the book, and in that one special moment, you've made a serious commitment to each other.

By removing a page right in front of you, your lover has just given a promise that, no matter what, *you are going to be seduced* in a fresh, exciting, original, and highly erotic manner. Sometime during the week, *your sensual pleasure* will be the only focus. You, of course, are making the same promise in return.

And neither of you has any idea what the other is planning! The pages are sealed, in fact, and you have to read yours in private. Each one contains a complete seduction, written out step-by-delicious, detailed step. Some of them are simple, fast, and fun —"quickies" designed to startle and excite your lover. If you've ever felt like sex was getting too predictable, just wait until you get to Seduction number… well, I think I'll keep that a secret for now, too.

On the other hand, some of these scenarios require a bit of planning. You might spend hours setting it up just right, and the end result will be absolutely unforgettable. There is nothing in the world quite so thrilling as the thought that someone went to a whole lot of effort to make you feel special. And best of all—*you get all the credit!* Remember, these recipes for great sex are a secret, so your partner will never know which ideas came from the book…and which were fueled by your own steamy and slightly naughty imagination.

And let's hope some recent recreational reading has helped fuel your imagination. The world has been electrified and energized by E.L. James' *Fifty Shades of Grey* trilogy and a few seductions here—*that I wrote about even before I read the novels*—will sound very familiar. Have fun with them as you get the chance to be Anastasia Steele and Christian Grey for the night!

You'll eventually notice some common threads linking these seductions, and here's one of the most important: almost all of them ask you to do something to *tease your lover.* Often it's just a hint; the tiniest little clue left lying about early in the week to remind your bedmate of the surprise in store. Now, if you find a seduction that's not exactly your cup a tea, feel free to change it. I'll bet you can come up with something that suits you even better. But please— please!—*keep that element of anticipation.* It's the heart and soul of this book. That sense of expectancy is more than just spice in the sauce. It's what elevates sex from mundane to magnificent. It transforms intercourse from an athletic event into one of the mysteries of the universe.

And, because of this, no matter how stressed or strapped for time you are, you'll *find* the time to carry it out. You'll come to covet these special moments together, especially since these seductions were created to give each of you *exactly what you're looking for*—that is, if you're anything like the thousands of people I've talked to over the years.

On hundreds of radio and TV shows across the country, as I was researching and promoting some of my nine books on the subject, I heard what men and women want in the bedroom. We want to know how to turn our mates on. We want them to know what turns us on. We'd like more variety... more foreplay... more surprises... more interest...new tricks... and once in a while, somebody *else* should do all the work! And that's what gave me the idea for this book:

Fifty seductions written for *his* eyes only, spelling out exactly how to get her attention, how to make her laugh, how to make her want you–and how to bring her to new heights of passion.

Fifty seductions written for *her* eyes only, filled with clever and fun ways to spark his interest, each with an unusual twist or *advanced sexual technique* designed to fan that spark into a white-hot flame.

And finally, **one very special seduction to be read by both of you**. Number 101 is a sort of graduation exercise for my newest Masters of The Erotic Arts—save this one for last.

Welcome To The New 2020 Edition!

So much has happened since publishing the last edition of this book: I have spent the last several years immersing myself in the business of sex, now more exciting than ever in our highly charged world, and I've been working with a lot of great experts and writers in the field, from Gwyneth Paltrow—I had the honor of joining forces with her and Goop to contribute to their book, The Sex Issue—to Anna del Gaizo, also known as the Playboy Advisor, to writer and journalist Stephanie Theobald, whose work explores the lines beyond sexual boundaries.

Speaking of which, I've also discovered a number of great books on the topic of sex: *Pussy: A Reclamation* by Regina Thomashauer should be required reading for all women, Esther Perel's *Mating in Captivity* is a groundbreaking work on how to keep the fire alive in long term relationships, and Theobald's *Sex Drive: On the Road to a Pleasure Revolution* is a must-read guide for repossessing your sex drive. From the classic *The 5 Love Languages* to the innovative *She Comes First* to the change-effecting *Love Worth Making* to yes, Goop's *The Sex Issue*, with over a thousand books in my library, I love to do my research and then take those fresh ideas to test out in my bedroom! You'll find inspiring tidbits from all these books inside the sealed envelopes.

You'll also find lots of fun new seductions, including the deliciously playful Cherry Lips; life-changing Queen V, featuring sex education pioneer Betty Dodson; and epic Best.One.Ever. (Make sure you rip that one out! You'll want to hear the story of how a single photo revolutionized my sex life forever—and how you can snap one of your own.)

Celebrities like Britney Spears, Sharon Stone, Ryan Seacrest, and the ladies of *The View* have all been inspired to rip open my sealed envelopes, and they've loved the results. While I might be known as the Sex Coach to the Stars, I'm really here for you. We all need a little permission sometimes to come out and play.

For the past twenty-five years, I've discussed these seductions with people from across the country—couples who've used these techniques to put the sexual excitement back into their relationships. I've heard which erotic encounters have worked best for them. They've also been kind enough to share with me how they've improved upon their favorites and altered them to fit their needs. Thanks to their contributions, I've been able to add their ideas and enhancements to this new edition and I can't close this introduction without a word of thanks to these readers.

I'm thrilled to be updating *101 Nights of Great Sex* because trends are always changing and you can always do more to improve your sex life. But one thing never changes: the anticipation of an erotic encounter, plus the surprises you spring on your partner, plus the excitement of the seduction itself, plus the thrill of trying new things with your lover—it all adds up to truly Great Sex. Don't just read about it. Do it! And thank me later.

Laura Corn
Santa Monica, California

Now – some final notes before you start your big adventure:

Hygiene. It's critical! I can't tell you how many men and women have told me they've lost interest in sex because their partner has some personal grooming flaws. Think of it this way—as you go through this book, your lover is going to kiss and nibble and lick and suck various parts of you, *a lot*! You're going to do the same. Fresh breath, clean teeth, shampooed hair, and scrubbed skin—it's the uniform you put on *before* the game of love.

Money. Most of these seductions cost nothing at all. But for those that do, I've included little icons on the title pages to give you an idea of what to expect.

No $ at all mean it's free, or under ten dollars.

$ means 10 to 25 dollars.

$$ means 30 to 60 dollars.

$$$ means 65 to 100 dollars.

100+   means over a hundred dollars.

Yes, there are even a couple that cost a lot—if your budget permits, the sky's the limit. And yes, I think you should plan one or two seductions every year where you pull out all the stops! Anniversaries, Birthdays, Valentine's Day, etc… what you're buying are memories that will last a lifetime.

The rest of the icons. The road means you're going somewhere. The cherry indicates food is involved. The mask means that there are toys involved. The envelope indicates a Teaser has been created especially for this seduction. This extra treat can be sent to your lover from www.101Nights.com and is optional. For a more detailed description of these icons, please see the Icon Guide page.

Props. Lots of these seductions encourage you to buy extra little items to dress up the event. Most are inexpensive and easy to find, and to help you locate any that aren't available in your town, I've included a list of websites and mail-order catalogs on the Laura Corn product page. Don't just ignore these special ingredients! It's extra touches like these that convince your sweetheart that you really mean it. If you can't find what I've suggested, *substitute*. Use your imagination. It really is the effort that counts.

Laura Corn, I just CAN'T do that! Yes, you can. Sooner or later, especially if you're a shy person, chances are you'll come across a seduction that seems too wild or too extravagant or simply too much for you. I say—just do it! Do it, do it, do it! Almost a million other couples have, so please give it a try. Your partner might be thrilled. You might learn to love something new. And if you can't, well, at least don't give up on your promise to your mate. Pull out another seduction... or make up one of your own. The important thing is to make your partner's pleasure a top priority at least once a week.

Did I mention GREAT sex? That is, of course, only if you finish this introduction, grab your partner, and start tearing out the pages. So go on—start right now. My job is done.

You, on the other hand, are just beginning. It's a one-year course in the ancient art of seduction, and when you're done, you'll have one tattered, empty book cover...

And a lot of *great memories*.

Enjoy!

SEDUCTION AND ICON GUIDE

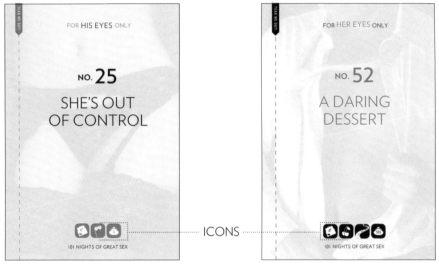

FOR **HIS EYES** ONLY

NO. 25

SHE'S OUT
OF CONTROL

101 NIGHTS OF GREAT SEX

FOR **HER EYES** ONLY

NO. 52

A DARING
DESSERT

101 NIGHTS OF GREAT SEX

ICONS

FOR **HIS EYES** ONLY

FOR **HER EYES** ONLY

 Teaser

 Involves Food

 Involves Toys

 Going Somewhere

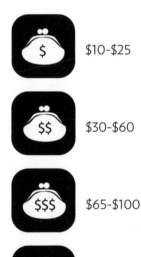

$10-$25

$30-$60

$65-$100

over $100

FOR **HIS EYES** ONLY

NO. **1**

HONEYLINGUS

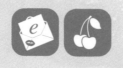

101 NIGHTS OF GREAT SEX

The ingredients might already be in your own home, and if not, it's easy to find a quart of milk and a small squeeze jar of honey. Tie them together with a ribbon or string, and attach a note to them in the fridge: "Don't touch! I have a surprise for you this week!" Promise her a surprise, create some romantic anticipation, and you're halfway to Great Sex already. Pick a night when you're staying in, and offer to draw a bath for her. Add three or four cups of milk to create a special treat, an *exfoliant milk bath*.

Be sure to set a romantic scene for her, with candles in the bathroom and music on the stereo. And make sure to get an old washable blanket and lay it across your bed. Trust me on this, she'll be much more relaxed if she knows she won't have to clean up a big mess afterwards.

As she finishes her bath, bring her the honey and offer her a proposition. "I want to play a little game with you. After I leave the bathroom, I want you to hide six dabs of honey anywhere on your body. Anywhere at all," you say, "kind of like this." Squeeze a few drops on the side of her neck, just above her collarbone. Don't let it run; instead, rub it with your fingertip into a small, sticky circle.

"And then," you continue, "I'm going to try to find them all. Like this." Lean in and lick it off, *suck* it off, nibble it off, and just in case you missed some, move up to her ear, and the back of her neck, gently nuzzling and kissing her everywhere you go. Make it perfectly clear that you expect to give your tongue a real workout tonight. "Remember, six little dabs. Hide them anywhere, front and back, and then come join me in the bedroom."

Find your honey's honey. Connect the dots with your tongue. Work the areas that don't usually get enough attention. Knees and toes, shoulders and wrists, breasts, nipples, thighs, bum; pay them all a visit. Finally, of course, you need to focus on your real goal, your honeypie's Honeypot. And at this point, you should take your cue from my new bar friend, the one with the amazing China tale:

Every story needs a *dàtuányuán*. (A happy ending!)

NO.1 HONEYLINGUS

INGREDIENTS

1 quart of milk

1 squeezable bottle of honey

1 blanket, washable, to protect your bed sheets

1 strong tongue

1 Note (with string or ribbon)

I COULD HARDLY BELIEVE MY LUCK. A girlfriend and I were sitting at the bar of a beautiful restaurant in LA when I found myself face-to-face with a famous rock star. I might have been a tiny bit starstruck. After all, I used to save my allowance to buy his music, and here he was, talking to me.

Sadly, I didn't learn anything about him that you couldn't read for yourself on Wikipedia. But his *friend*—now here was a guy who had a fascinating tale to tell. Not only was he rich and devilishly handsome but he'd also lived a bachelor's dream, and had been with thousands of women around the world. I couldn't help myself. I just had to ask. "What would you say is the best sex you've ever had?"

Without hesitation, he answered, "The Milk and Honey Massage, in Beijing, China"—the most erotic massage technique I have ever heard of. It involved milk and honey, slathered on with a soft brush, and then lovingly removed with an exceedingly thorough tongue bath. Wow. I wanted my *own* Milk and Honey Massage!

I knew my readers would want one, too, so I took the idea home and finally came up with a recipe any man can follow. Yes, it involves milk and honey, but at its core, this technique is about *attention*. Complete, total focus on your partner's sensual pleasure. Sexual service + romance + a killer skin conditioning treatment = every woman's dream! (And it costs practically nothing. Seriously, dollars to orgasms, it's the best value in the book.)

SEND HER THE TEASER!

TYPE THE LINK BELOW. CASE SENSITIVE.

101nights.com/
Honeylingus

FOR HER EYES ONLY

NO. 2

THE VELVET
TONGUE

101 NIGHTS OF GREAT SEX

to sit down on the edge of the bed with his feet on the floor, your drink in hand. If you want to push it a step further, blindfold him beforehand so he doesn't know where all that warm, sexy magic is coming from – a little bewilderment can make for a great tease! Take a sip, generous enough for it to make an impact but not so much that liquid will pour out of your mouth, and don't swallow. Place the mug on your bedside table for quick access.

Then plant a kiss deep on his lips. Explore the inside of his mouth with your hot tongue. Run it across his teeth and back over his lips. Explore the inside of his mouth with your hot tongue. Nibble his neck, then — after a quick sip to keep the steam up — pull his nipples into your mouth. Don't be afraid to bite. Gently, of course...

Work your way down to his stomach, and when you get to his penis, completely soak it in wet heat. Lick it — top to bottom, front to back. Pull his scrotum into your mouth, and let your tongue trace the out-line of his testicles. Take another sip and run your tongue up and down his frenulum, that super-sensitive area where the shaft meets the head. Heat engorges a man's penis—just the opposite effect of a cold shower—so don't be surprised if he's bigger than ever. Speaking of surprises, I should warn you: a mouthful of hot liquid will also speed up his orgasm and make it twice as intense.

And twice as addictive.

NO. 2 THE VELVET TONGUE

INGREDIENTS

plain hot water or hot beverage of your choice

1 naked man

1 soft wet tongue

TIMELESS, STRIPPED-DOWN AND STRAIGHT-UP sexy: Some of the best seductions are classics, only requiring a bare essential or two. Years ago, one of my all-time favorite techniques came to national attention, thanks to *The Late Show with David Letterman* and his then-guest Heather Locklear. Dave asked her what she'd been doing lately and before my astonished eyes, she said she'd been going through this really hot book, *101 Nights of Great Sex*. That's right: the original edition of *this* book. As the audience whooped and cheered, Heather responded, "Oh, so you guys have heard of it. I especially love the Velvet Tongue."

Me too! Me too! Now over two-and-a-half decades later, this enduring gem has satisfied millions of men – and made heroes of just as many women.

The key ingredient to the Velvet Tongue is a warm drink. It's that simple. Chamomile tea, spiced cider: Take your pick, though I find a cup of hot coffee works best for me. Start off by asking him

SEND HIM THE TEASER!

TYPE THE LINK BELOW. CASE SENSITIVE.

101nights.com/
TheVelvetTongue

FOR HER EYES ONLY

NO. 3

SHAKE & BAKE

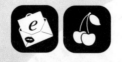

101 NIGHTS OF GREAT SEX

Send him a text while he's at work. *Hey, babe. Making you something special for dinner.* Don't reveal that there's anything else going on. When he gets home and you come out in only your apron and your heels, pretend that it's no big deal. You always cook like this, right?

Is he watching? You bet he is. You've got his attention in a way that the football game never will. So, play it up to the fullest. Bend toward him and let your breasts shake a little while you chop veggies. Run an ice cube over your neck and then suck on it saying, "I always get so hot when I cook." Every time you open the oven (which should be often), make sure your butt's in the air. Taste everything slowly, leisurely, and with sound effects. *Mm-mm. This is sooo good.*

Pretty soon, he'll be right there in the kitchen with you. He can only stand to watch you shake your butt and wiggle your breasts for so long before he's going to want to touch you. Let him touch, but only a little. Remind him that too much snacking will ruin his appetite.

Tease him by asking, "*Is this spicy enough?*" Offer him your finger (or another body part) to taste. It never hurts to spill a drop or two of something. Maybe it falls on the inside of your arm. Or on your belly. Or down between your breasts. Let him lick it off. If some gets on your apron, no worries. Just slide out of it and show him all the other places you might have spilled something. Along your nipples. Between your thighs... now, how did that get there?

All this nibbling and tasting is going to make him so hungry for you that he won't be able to wait. So let him eat you up. Life's too short not to have dessert first.

NO.3 SHAKE & BAKE

INGREDIENTS

1 recipe that's easy to cook

all recipe ingredients

1 sexy apron (available at jessiesteele.com)

high heels

THEY SAY THE WAY TO A MAN'S HEART is through his stomach. But the way to a man's libido is through his eyes. The truth is, no matter how we feel about our bodies, he thinks we're hot as hell. Especially when we're doing something domestic.

Especially when we're doing it in the nude—or nearly nude.

You're going to fulfill one of your man's biggest fantasies by feeding both his heart and his lust. That's right: You're going to become your very own version of the naked chef. With a little extra dash of spice.

The special seasoning for this seduction is the *apron*. Aprons are the perfect peek-a-boo clothing, whether they're see-through, skimpy and tied around the waist to show off your gorgeous breasts, or full-body aprons that offer just a glimpse of hips and butt once you turn around. Heels are the garnish, as they lengthen your legs and highlight your calves.

Plus, they make that perfect click-clack across the kitchen floor that gives men instant hard-ons.

SEND HIM THE TEASER!

TYPE THE LINK BELOW. CASE SENSITIVE.

101nights.com/
ShakeandBake

FOR **HIS EYES** ONLY

NO. **4**

MASSAGE
COLLAGE

As soon as she reads your text, she's going to be enticed. Intrigued. Most of all, excited. She's feeling teased in the best way possible and she now has a day or two for the suspense to build. Part one of your mission is already accomplished. Part two is even better.

What is it about towels and robes that have just come out of the dryer? Maybe they pick up some sort of magic in there, because every woman is transported to a happier place as soon as she wraps herself up in them. But that's nothing compared to the happy place *you're* about to take her.

Start your Saturday Night sex date with a regular massage, with her facing down on the bed. Warm room, soft music, flickering candles. Work her shoulders like a pro…but kiss her neck like a lover. Rub her feet with hot oil…but straddle her thighs while you do it, so she can feel your erection growing. But don't rush into sex just yet — you want to give her time to think about it while she's enjoying her massage.

Gradually raise the stakes. Let your hands roam where no professional would go. Keep kneading her muscles, but let your swelling penis glide between her thighs and press up against her outer lips. Slip it inside, but only a few inches, and for only a few strokes. Pull out, and keep massaging her back. A minute later, pull her legs apart and slip back in. This time, let her feel your weight and a firm thrust…then pull out and continue rubbing her back.

Then do it all again.

Take your time, alternating between massage, tongue, and penis, pushing her up through layer after layer of stimulation. Keep going until she's standing right on that precious, blissful edge of orgasm.

Then push her over. You're gonna love the ride down.

NO. 4 MASSAGE COLLAGE

INGREDIENTS

1 bottle of massage oil

candles

sexy music

dryer full of warm towels
and a bathrobe

1 hot shower

FOR A WOMAN, THIS IS FANTASY SEX. Dream sex. Ultimate sex.

Don't worry, your turn is coming. And it'll be an all-out circus complete with blowjobs, I promise. Real guy sex. But this week you're going to give your woman the kind of erotic experience she would buy for herself, if she were that kind of gal. Actually, it's the kind of sex she's secretly wishing for every time she goes to a luxury spa. Call girls even have a name for it: *Massage...with release.* That'll be a hundred dollars, please.

Tonight's erotic play starts with a tease a few days ahead of time. Send her a text that says something like this:

> **What's better than a massage?**
>
> *You're going to find out this weekend.*
>
> **Saturday Night's agenda:**
>
> *7:15 Relaxing, candlelit bath (just for you)*
>
> *7:45 Warm towels, warm robe*
>
> *8:00 Massage*
>
> *8:15 Massage Collage*
>
> **Sunday's agenda:**
>
> *Recover*

SEND HER THE TEASER!

TYPE THE LINK BELOW. CASE SENSITIVE.

101nights.com/
MassageCollage

FOR HER EYES ONLY

NO. 5

I'M SO
BUZZED

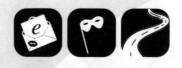

101 NIGHTS OF GREAT SEX

He might ask if the fridge is broken again, or if the dryer is acting up, or, or… *"Here's a little hint,"* you interrupt him. Then put the phone down near your waist for a couple of seconds so he can hear the buzzing sound of your vibrator. *"Does that sound familiar?"* By now he knows that sound, or should. Tell him, *"Oh, I think I found the problem. I'll call you right back!"* Then hang up.

Two minutes later, call him in his car. Put the phone between your thighs, and let him listen for a moment. Yes, it is. It's your vibrator, humming happily along. Tell him all about it. Tell him how hot you are. Tell him you're right on the edge, but you're waiting for him to come home and help you finish. Tell him to hurry because things are heating up and you're feeling lonely for his love. Let him listen for another few seconds, then hang up and wait.

You won't have to wait long. He's going to *fly* home, with a bone in his britches. And when he comes stumbling into the bedroom, he'll see exactly what he's been imagining for the last few miles. You'll be nearly naked, with your legs spread wide, face flushed, a sheen of sexy sweat on your skin. And a vibrator held tight against your mound. After ten minutes of torture in traffic, this blissfully erotic image will be seared into his brain for a long long time.

Call him over to the bed. Hand him the toy and tell him to take over and hold it snug against you, while you open his pants and pull out his erect penis. You need something firm to grab on to because, after ten minutes of struggling *not* to give in to the power of the vibe, you, my lady, are about to go flying.

I'M SO BUZZED

INGREDIENTS

2 cell phones

1 loud vibrator
(I recommend the classic old school "Magic Wand" vibrator. Gentle enough for the lady bits and strong enough for his.)

HIGHWAYS. BUSES. TRAINS AND SUBWAYS. They were invented to make life easier and faster for all of us, but the long, boring commute can sometimes make you want to tear your hair out— the crowded stations, the buses with no seats left, the endless red lights!

But not for your guy, not this week. Thanks to a couple of other modern inventions that we've come to take for granted, you are going to make his drive home positively thrilling. Set up the commute of his life by giving him a mysterious instruction in the morning: *He must call you when he is ten minutes from home.* Why? Oh, you've got a surprise for him. A big surprise. That's all he needs to know. Call or text him during the day to remind him—*call when you're ten minutes away.*

When he rings you at home, your conversation will sound something like this—

> Him: *"What's up?"*

> You: *"I need your help, baby. I have a little mechanical issue that needs your attention."*

SEND HIM THE TEASER!

TYPE THE LINK BELOW. CASE SENSITIVE.

101nights.com/
ImSoBuzzed

FOR HER EYES ONLY

NO. **6**

DIAMOND
GIRL

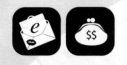

because women instinctively know it looks sexy, and men consistently forget to breathe when they see it. Jewelry on bare skin is, I dare say, the reason why men buy jewelry. If your guy doesn't always seem to notice your jewelry, it's simply because your clothes get in the way.

With this information in mind, you can create a scene of jaw-dropping beauty and sensuality for your lover. First, get undressed and put on all your best jewelry. Choose it carefully: a crystal-encrusted choker, single strand of pearls, a twinkling ring or delicate anklet. When it comes to earrings, the bigger, the better. Use your discretion when it comes to layering; the idea is just enough, not jangling to the point of distraction. You want to save the spotlight for the real focal point: a nipple-and-clit clamp. If you've never bought one, or seen one, for that matter, head to UnboundBabes.com and snap one up. And if this final accessory seems a little extreme, it is—*in the best way possible*. The moment you put it on, you'll feel like pure sex. The only other thing you should wear is a pair of your most ruthlessly sexy high heels.

Line your bedroom with candles. Lots of them. Pile pillows on your bed and kneel on top of them. Call your lover to the room. Watch his mouth fall open.

In that sensuous candlelight, with sparkling gems and sexy stilettos adorning you, his eyes will pop out of his head. That's because you look amazing. Elegant. Glorious. Shamelessly sexy. You're a cross between a showgirl and a princess. (Oh! Do you know where to find a tiara?) Tonight, you are making your lover feel like a very, very rich man, in every sense of the word.

Now take him to bed. Let him feel the cool metal of your gems against his own bare skin. Let him see how your ears, your belly, and your breasts dazzle. How your jewels and your lips glisten in the light. Let him hear the erotic jangle of your accessories as you climb on him, or thrust against him, or bob your head up and down on him. Finish him off. And then, just to show him what jewelry can do for a woman, finish him off again.

Forget breakfast at Tiffany's—you've just earned yourself a whole day there. Time to put a little ding on the credit card!

NO.6 DIAMOND GIRL

INGREDIENTS

pieces of your
favorite jewelry

nipple-and-clit
body chain
(unboundbabes.
com)

high heels

candles

*"If I had my way, I'd wear jewelry, a great
pair of heels and nothing else."*

JADA PINKETT SMITH

I'm with you, Jada! Wearing jewelry doesn't feel
great just because it's pretty or sentimental. There's
potency in adorning your body, letting yourself
gleam and glisten like a powerful goddess. You
probably think your guy doesn't even notice your
jewelry. But it isn't true.

And here's how I know. While writing my first
book, *237 Intimate Questions Every Woman Should
Ask A Man*, I interviewed over one thousand men
and asked them this question:

> "If a woman were to do a long, slow,
> sensuous striptease for you and just leave
> on two things…what would they be?"
> And the number one answer was: shoes
> and earrings! See, they *do* like it when we
> wear sparkly stuff. (And they like it even
> better when that is all we wear.)

In fact, a quick trip to your local museum or
a glance at an art book—especially a book of
tasteful erotic images—and you'll be convinced.
Many classic paintings and eye-catching images
show women who are *not quite* nude. Instead,
they are posing with precious stones and bangles,
gold hoops and bracelets, and loop after loop of
pearls set against nakedness. It's a look that is as
old as jewelry itself. It will *never* go out of fashion,

SEND HIM
THE TEASER!

TYPE THE LINK BELOW. CASE SENSITIVE.

101nights.com/
DiamondGirl

FOR **HIS EYES** ONLY

NO. 7

BANG FOR THE BUCK

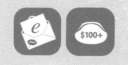

101 NIGHTS OF GREAT SEX

On your special day, tuck the necklace into the nightstand drawer, or under your pillow. Make sure it's hidden, but accessible from the bed. You'll also need a soft scarf or a blindfold. Now, go out and enjoy your evening. Wine and dine. Romance and flirt. Build that electricity with every touch, so you both know when you get home, sparks are gonna fly.

Once you're in the bedroom, kissing, touching, and undressing (you've got this part, right?) pull out the blindfold, and cover her eyes. Kiss her cheeks, the nape of her neck, her throat and her collar bone. Take your time. Let her simmer. Quietly pull the necklace from its hiding place as you lean her over the bed or a nearby chair. You're going to take her from behind, while she's blindfolded.

Now choose your moment as you're pumping inside her. Slow down. Slip the necklace around her neck and work the clasp. Let the weight of it fall against her throat, tracing the precious metal with your fingertips. Tell her how amazing she looks as you resume your thrusts, pushing her toward climax...

When you finally collapse together onto the bed in a tangle of arms and legs, remove the blindfold and catch your breath.

She's gonna want to see the necklace of course, so take her by the hand and lead her to the mirror. Put your arms around her and let her gaze at the two of you there, with the flush of orgasm coloring her cheeks and the beautiful necklace shimmering along her collarbone, tell her how incredible she really is.

You've done it—*forever imprinted in her heart and mind a powerful link between this amazing night of mind-blowing sex and the beautiful necklace around her neck.*

Now every time she wears this necklace, catching sight of it in every mirror, the image is gonna make her smile. In fact, I'll bet the image triggers more than her memory.

Are you ready for a repeat performance?

NO.7 BANG FOR THE BUCK

INGREDIENTS

4 electric candles

1 scarf or blindfold

1 dinner reservation or plan a meal at home

1 special necklace. (It could be a choker, or a necklace with a pendant. Shashi and Argento Vivo are both affordable brands sold on Amazon. You can also find a Tiffany necklace on Google for under $150. Every woman loves Tiffany!)

WHEN A WOMAN RECEIVES THE GIFT OF JEWELRY she remembers everything about that moment. The time of day, where she was, what she was wearing, what he was wearing—every detail is seared into her memory. You've seen it in commercials, the little velvet box, the flickering candlelight, and that magic moment when she opens the lid and gasps in surprise. And the best news is jewelry doesn't have to be expensive to have that effect.

Imprinting is a powerful thing, forging a connection that lasts a lifetime. Now, imagine harnessing that power, and using it for good! This week, you're gonna imprint her heart and mind forever, with a gift of jewelry...*during sex*.

That's right...right in the middle of lovemaking, you're gonna surprise her with a necklace, and create a mind blowing memory, an imprint unlike anything she's ever experienced. Send her a little text early in the week. Tell her you love her, she's incredible, and hot, and you can't imagine life without her. If words aren't your thing, ask Hallmark for help. You know her favorite restaurant, or maybe you want to cook for her. Either way, make her an invite to dinner she can't refuse.

Next, you've got some shopping to do. You want a lovely necklace, that she'll want to wear often— a delicate pendant on a chain, perhaps a silver choker. Check out her jewelry box, if you need a sense of what she likes.

SEND HER THE TEASER!

TYPE THE LINK BELOW. CASE SENSITIVE.

101nights.com/ BangForTheBuck

FOR **HIS EYES** ONLY

NO. **8**

CLIT BAIT

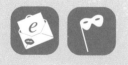

101 NIGHTS OF GREAT SEX

Are there any other toys you've tried that she loves? Throw them in. The point is, use your imagination to spark hers. Then close the lid and tape it shut. (Interesting side note: This may be the only time in your entire life you employ duct tape for the purpose of seduction.)

Friday morning, hand her the box. "This," you say with a smile, "can give you the greatest orgasm you've ever had." Umm...what did you just say? "You heard me. Best orgasm ever. In this box. Wanna know what it is?"

Well, yeah, she does want to know. She wants to know pretty bad, in fact. But she can't open it, not until Saturday night. And that means for almost two whole days, she'll be thinking about that orgasm and imagining what's in the box. She'll shake it. She'll move it around. And no matter what else she does, she'll always find her thoughts drifting back to that box.

Come Friday night, send her the Tease! Like a kid the night before Christmas, she won't be able to sleep – but she also won't care. Her excitement levels are through the roof!

On Saturday evening, tell her to bring the mysterious box to the bedroom. Dim the lights, put on some sexy music, and unseal the box. But before you open it... blindfold her (use something soft and silky). A satin sleep mask works; so does one of your ties. And then, one by one, pull your surprises from the box. Use them. And use your hands and mouth and everything else. Stimulate her sense of touch, her sense of smell, her sense of taste. But the real object tonight is to overwhelm that one sense that's been on edge for days, like an erotic itch just begging to be scratched:

Her sense of anticipation.

Congratulations. You've just mastered the art of Clit Bait!

NO. 8 CLIT BAIT

INGREDIENTS

1 box (a nice shoebox or any box will do)

tape

massage oil

music

1 scented candle

1 vibrator

1 blindfold

assorted playthings (hit up your favorite adult store and pick up a feather tickler, cute spanking paddle or mini leather whip, a pair of pretty handcuffs, something lacy for her to wear and so on)

IF YOU'VE GOT A BOX, YOU CAN TURN ANY WOMAN ON.

No, seriously. No one loves an expensive gift more than me, but I have to share one of the Great Truths of Great Sex: Diamonds aren't really a girl's best friend. What really makes a woman hot is not jewelry, or flowers, or anything you can buy. It's not even romance. (But this doesn't mean you can skip the jewels, flowers and romance!)

No, what makes an orgasm great — earth-shattering, mind-blowing, out-of-this-world great — is anticipation. Hey, sex is good, pretty much any time. But you know what's even better? Sex you've been thinking about. Sex you've been waiting for, and dreaming of, and planning. For a woman, the act of imagining sex counts as foreplay, and when it comes to foreplay, here's Laura's number one rule: More is better.

Which brings me back to the box and how you can use it to get your woman hot. Start by filling it with some of her favorite sex stuff. Massage oil, of course. A brand-new dildo. Fresh tube of lipstick. And plenty of hot surprises: neon-pink bondage tape. A necklace featuring a vibrator pendant. Rainbow-hued pinwheel. Nipple tats or pasties. And a skiers hand-warmer (that's right, you'll want to use it to rub on her pubic bone while you lick her for an amazing sensation she won't forget).

SEND HER THE TEASER!

TYPE THE LINK BELOW. CASE SENSITIVE.

101nights.com/ClitBait

FOR HER EYES ONLY

NO. 9

CHERRY
LIPS

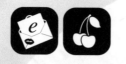

101 NIGHTS OF GREAT SEX

TEAR ME OUT!

inner Roller Girl, skates or barefoot. These are all extras. The pièce de résistance here is your ice-cold popsicle – and you, all doe-eyed and hot and bothered.

Speaking of hot, have the heat cranked up just a little higher than normal. (Don't make it sweltering, though. Most men like to be on the cooler side.) Just enough to make him want to get out of his clothes as soon as he gets home. Be ready when he approaches, so you can greet him at the door. When you do, he'll find you, licking a popsicle as if it's no big deal with a great big smile on your face. You can bet he'll be grinning ear-to-ear by now too, too.

"What are you up to?!" he'll probably say. *"Oh, I just had a hankering for a popsicle. Want some?"* Draw it to his lips so he can have a taste, before you take it back and start tantalizing him with it. Wrap your red-stained lips around it. The cherry-colored hue is going to bring him back to adolescence; when he was young, carefree and the sight of a girl sucking on something would make his head spin. Lick it up and down. *"Mmm!"* Keep your icy stick in one hand and start tugging his clothes off with the other, as you lead him to the bedroom. Once you're there, pull down his pants. Trace your fingertips along his penis until he's rock-hard and then take another suck on your pop. It's probably starting to melt a little by now, and that's a good thing. Get messy, get sticky; rub it in between your breasts in between licks. Now you want to start licking *him*.

The cold sensation on him will probably come as a shock, but the heat of your mouth is going to create a mind-blowing combination. Note: The longer you keep the popsicle in your mouth, the colder your tongue becomes. And the redder it gets! Which is what this icy oral treat is all about. When he sees your plump, red-stained lips wrapped around his shaft, it will blow his mind. Give him *looong* licks with your cherry tongue, like his penis is that popsicle! You've been teasing him since he got home, and now he finally gets the ultimate treat; your luscious red lips and tongue going to town on him.

Get into a rhythm and don't be afraid to giggle as you come up for air. Good humor is everything! Once you're so worked up you can't take it anymore, or once your treat has disappeared down to it's wooden stick, slowly climb on top of him and ride him just like you know Roller Girl would.

NO. 9 CHERRY LIPS

INGREDIENTS

1 cherry popsicle

1 sexy swimsuit

1 babysitter as needed

IS THERE ANYTHING MORE REFRESHING THAN an ice-cold popsicle on a hot summer day? Maybe you haven't had one since you were a little girl. Do you remember running cherry-flavored pops over your lips to create a nice red stain? Well, now you're going to use the frozen treat to create something as naughty as it is nice! This seduction is one-part nostalgia and two-parts innocence with one big helping of all-American sex appeal.

It doesn't matter what the temperature is outside, although this will be especially enticing on a sultry day. Pick a time when nobody else will be home; you'll want the privacy! In the middle of the day, you're going to send him a text letting him know there's a heatwave about to happen: *Baby, I'm so hot. You're going to need to help cool me off when you get home.* Let him be a little confused. He'll know *exactly* what's going on soon enough.

Now it's time to get ready. Put on your favorite bikini (extra points if it's in a cute bright color) or something summery, like a tight tank top and pair of terry-cloth shorts. Pull your hair into a high ponytail and rub a hint of berry-colored stain on your lips. Maybe add a coat of mascara but no other makeup: You're an ingenue...who's ready to lose her chastity!

If you happen to have a pair of roller skates buried in your closet, this is the time to bring them out! Finally, put on some retro music: "Hot Child in the City" by Nick Gilder or "Brand New Key" by Melanie. Actually, the whole *Boogie Nights* soundtrack will help you get in touch with your

SEND HIM
THE TEASER!

TYPE THE LINK BELOW. CASE SENSITIVE.

101nights.com/CherryLips

FOR **HIS EYES** ONLY

NO. 10

MAKE HER TREMBLE

perfect for this shower surprise. It's light and easy to handle in the water, and it doesn't completely block out light. She will squirm with delight as you wrap the gauze slowly around her eyes. She'll still sense the flickering of the candles in the dim room. But it moves her one step further from reality, and another step away from control.

The second surprise is a lovely, fresh aroma. Don't tell her what it is. Just step in the shower and let her smell your bottle of ultra-rich, moisturizing in-shower body lotion. It's not soap; it's a special lotion that goes on in the shower, and it's smooth and slippery and smells like heaven. Use it like massage oil. Apply it to her hot, wet skin and rub it in. Concentrate on the muscles of her shoulders and neck.

And now, for surprise number three. Just outside the shower, you hid a cup of ice. By now, the ice cubes have melted into smooth, round chips. Reach out of the shower, pick up a small ice cube, and press it against your lover's skin while she is still standing under the stream of hot water. *Gasp!*

The ice is startling, but not painful, not in a steaming shower. Slide the cube along her skin. Play with it until it melts away. And then...pour out another handful of body lotion and spread it over her glistening skin. Just as she begins to relax, it's time for another touch of shocking cold, this time right under one breast. Draw the melting cube in a spiral right up to her nipple. After more wet heat, run another ice cube down her back, and between the cheeks of her bottom, and right through her thighs to her clitoris. Alternate, hot and cold, steam and frost. Her pulse is running faster, her breath a little shallower. She can barely see, so she's never quite sure what's coming next—more heat, more massage, or more chill. She's totally out of control now. She can do nothing but go along for the ride, and trust you to take her right to the edge of pleasure...

And push her over.

NO.10 MAKE HER TREMBLE

INGREDIENTS

1 shower

1 bottle of in-shower body lotion

1 cup of ice cubes

1 strip of cotton gauze (the kind used for bandages)

3 candles

THE MOST EXCITING THINGS in the world are, at their core, about *loss of control*. Roller coasters, falling in love, orgasms—they are thrilling because we can't stop them or steer them. Once they start, we can only go along for the ride, and hope we can catch our breath when they're over.

I dare you to take your sweetie on an erotic thrill ride this week. You already have the most critical ingredient—a shower—and the rest can be found at the drugstore for a few bucks.

Start by paying a little attention to her routine. It'll be worth it, trust me. Play private eye and figure out when it's a good night to get her hair wet (even if you're unaware, she's got a schedule for this sort of stuff). The day before, send her this text: *Things are about to get wet...you especially. Are you ready?* Of course she is! The next day, set out a few candles in the bathroom, turning on the shower to a perfectly steamy temperature and hide the rest of the supplies. Then the follow-up text: *I've got a surprise for you, but you have to get in the shower first. Come on in, sexy.* Lead her into the bathroom and let her soak under the hot spray while you prepare the rest of your surprises.

The first is a blindfold. It's actually just white cotton gauze, the kind used for first aid, and it's

SEND HER THE TEASER!

TYPE THE LINK BELOW. CASE SENSITIVE.

101nights.com/
MakeHerTremble

FOR **HIS EYES** ONLY

NO. **11**

POSITION OF SUBMISSION

101 NIGHTS OF GREAT SEX

attentiveness, and then move into some light wrestling. It's part of the build-up. Grab her waist with both your hands, lift her up, move her to exactly where you want her. Don't wait for her to get naked—strip her. No lovey-dovey talk tonight. Instead, tell her you think she's hot; tell her you're going to *do* her. Tell her to stand up, fingers laced behind her head, feet slightly apart, *now*. And just for emphasis, give her a little love-smack right on the ass.

Now play with her. Run your hands and your mouth over her body, and if she moves, remind her that you haven't given her permission yet. *Hmmm*, is another little spanking in order?

Order her into the Position of Submission: kneeling on the bed, bottom up, face down. Oh, yeah, you can have some fun here. You know where she keeps her vibrator, right? Hand it to her, and tell her to use it while you watch. It's a good thing her face is buried in the sheets, because she's lost in a fantasy—a sexual servant forced to perform for an audience. Let her press the toy against her clit for just a few moments, then...tell her to stop. Your turn again, to spank her, lick her, nip at her cheeks with your teeth. Order her to start with the vibe again, and watch as she gets wetter and wetter. Make her stop again; it's time for some more butt-play.

Mix up your commands so she's never quite sure what's coming next: a pop on the bum, or a ride on the toy. She's about to climax, but it's clear who's really in control of her orgasm. It's you.

And you're about to go for a ride yourself. Enter her from behind. Smack her bottom even harder, but now just with your hips as you pump in and out. Tell her to hold that vibrator hard against her clit, hard enough so that you can feel the tingle as it courses through her. And issue your final order:

Cum.

NO.11 POSITION OF SUBMISSION

INGREDIENTS

1 vibrator

1 set of balls

Head's Up!

This vibrator can also be used for Light Her Up, Clit Bait, Heels on a Dash, and Tongue & Cheek

"The perfect boyfriend is somebody who's really funny and easygoing but knows how to take control when needed. It's nice to have a man who can just tell you to calm down and chill out...and then throw you on the bed!"

MILLA JOVOVICH

Relationships are mostly about compromise. A little give-and-take keeps things running smoothly around the house. But when it comes to the bedroom, most women have a secret fantasy about a guy who's more take than give; a strong man who tells her what to do, and does what he wants. She doesn't want to *live* with that guy! He's kind of a jerk. But she does want to bang him every once in a while.

So this week, take command. Start by sending her the Tease, which will let her know things are about to get very physical, an enticing warning that she's going to get dominated—and she's going to like it. By the time the moment comes, she's going to be looking at you with a glint of anticipation in her eyes. She's wondering what's about to happen. Start by kissing her, with equal parts force and

SEND HER THE TEASER!

TYPE THE LINK BELOW. CASE SENSITIVE.

101nights.com/
PositionOfSubmission

FOR HER EYES ONLY

NO. 12

SEXY AF!

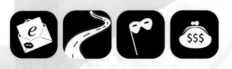

101 NIGHTS OF GREAT SEX

Awkward name aside, the whole buzz biz has come a long way. So buy a pair of remote control vibrating panties, or if you have your own lacy pair in mind you'd rather wear your own, pick up a remote control vibrator that comes with a magnetic clip to turn your Cosabella thong into your own private pleasure center (the Moxie by WeVibe is a good one). Then get ready to give your guy an unforgettable treat. You're going to let him turn you on. In public.

I strongly recommend that you test it once or twice before you take it outside. Maybe several times. You'll want to be familiar with exactly how it works. Then on a Saturday, pull on your electric–and now, electrifying!–underwear, get dressed, and ask your guy to take you on some errands.

While he's driving, hand him the remote control. You don't even have to explain. He'll figure it out. All he has to do is see the look on your face the first time he presses the remote control. Oh, yes, he knows that look. Turn it on: ecstasy. Turn it off: a happy dazed smile. It won't be long before he realizes what you've actually given him. It's more than just a cool toy, more than a wildly erotic experience. You've given him your trust. You've willfully given him command of your body, and that's a fantasy come true. You've taken on this techno-tease, now let him take control of your pleasure.

Things are about to get even more interesting. Stroll through the grocery store – the vegetable aisle is always fun! – and test out your new toy. Will it work when he's an aisle away? Can you walk with a vibe buzzing your clit? How many times can he bring you close to a climax? Can you keep a straight face? Can he?

The first time I tried this, I planned to let my honey tease me at stores all over town. I figured we would be buzzing at Starbuck's, humming in the drug store, zinging along the highways, tickling my kitty in Target, twitching as I ordered another drink on our night out. But guess what? I didn't make it past the checkout stand, and I'll bet you won't either. I predict you'll head for home, tear off those panties and jump into bed with your man.

(But will you make it? Or will you only get as far as the parking lot? Hmm. That sounds more like a dare...a double-A dare.)

NO.12 SEXY AF!

INGREDIENTS

1 silent remote control vibrating panty

1 (or more!) public places. (Grocery store, restaurant, park, nightclub)

I GUESS I WAS JUST AHEAD OF MY TIME.

Way back in 1999 I came across an amazing new gadget: the *remote controlled vibrator*. It was revolutionary, I thought, because it allowed couples to play together in ways that weren't possible before. That first model was bulky and noisy. But I knew that it was just the beginning of something big, and so I encouraged my readers to try it out.

Flash-forward to 2020. Clever, horny little minds have been busy stuffing the best of modern technology into the remote vibe. The newest versions come built into panties and are quiet enough to wear at the office. They're so small you can wear them under anything. The remote controls fit on a keychain, and the effect travels over a much longer distance. In fact—and I should have seen this coming—there are now panty-laced vibrators that require nothing more than a smartphone and WiFi connection. And that means supremely small, super-powered toys can be controlled from virtually anywhere on the planet. But trust me: You'll be grateful you're in close proximity to your partner once he takes over.

And you'll want to pick up one that comes with a remote control, no app necessary. No noise, no wires, no app store: just cyber waves of sheer pleasure. There's even a name for this *swelling* industry: Teledildonics. (Sigh. They're going to need a better name if they want to market this stuff to women. There's a reason they're far more commonly referred to as long-distance sex toys.)

SEND HIM THE TEASER!

TYPE THE LINK BELOW. CASE SENSITIVE.

101nights.com/SexyAF

NO. 13

COMING UNDONE

behind him…

Crrrack! I'll bet that's the first time he's been smacked on the ass with a belt in a long, long time. Laugh and let him have another. Smmmack! Hard enough to make him jump. Gentle enough to let him know it's all in good fun.

Now focus on that big, beautiful penis. Tease it with the belt. Slip it under his erection and lift it up, rubbing the hot skin and cool leather against your face. Grab his wrists and tie the belt around them in a loose knot. It doesn't have to be secure. Hey, he's not going anywhere: not with your mouth warming up the tip of his penis.

There are lots of ways to turn leather into foreplay. But the final move is yours, and it's one of my sexy favorites. Put the belt around your waist, leaving it loose and low. Take his hand and wrap his fingers around it. Whisper in his ear: "Hold on tight." Then turn around on your hands and knees, ass up high, belt slung under your hips. Aw yeah, that's hot. The belt gives him enough extra grip to pull you in closer and deeper and faster than ever before.

Everybody knows a belt is the best way to keep pants up. But for you two, it's also the fastest way to get them off.

INGREDIENTS

1 man's belt

YOUR MAN WALKS AROUND ALL DAY LONG with a sex toy in plain sight — how kinky! — and he doesn't even know it. It's his belt. And this Friday it's going to be the center of your erotic play.

On Monday, send him the Tease we created especially for this erotic encounter. It's just vague enough that it won't give anything away, but you can bet it will keep him thinking about you and your surprise all week long. Then ahead of your date, tell him to wear a belt. If he's not planning on it, change his mind: *You'll want to, trust me. You can thank me later.* When playtime rolls around, make a big show of removing his belt. Tug the buckle open slowly and slip the belt off, loop by loop. Drape it around the back of his neck, pull his face to yours, and give him a long, hard kiss.

Reach down and open his pants. Walk around him as you inch them down. Once you're standing

SEND HIM
THE TEASER!

TYPE THE LINK BELOW. CASE SENSITIVE.

101nights.com/
ComingUndone

FOR **HIS EYES** ONLY

NO.**14**

OMGYES!

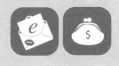

101 NIGHTS OF GREAT SEX

a woman's vagina. It may not look like the kind of raunchy shagging seen in Hollywood movies, but it's an area densely packed with nerves and it drives women craaaaaazy! This one included—OMG YES!

Send a text mid-week: *Sex ed class on Friday night. Take a shower and come to the bedroom at 8pm. Don't be late!*

Already she's intrigued.

On Friday morning, send her another text:

> Question: *What's the difference between a G-spot and a golf ball?*
>
> Answer: *A guy will actually search for a golf ball. BUT YOUR GUY IS GOING TO GO THE EXTRA MILE!!! Love from a lover who only wants to get better.*

That's going to make her smile and feel a whole lot of affection for you. Plus, a real G-spot orgasm? Wow, she thought they only existed in New York and LA!

On the big night, make sure you're showered and clean—and GET A MANICURE. Your fingers are going to be doing a lot of exploring, so they need to look good. Also make sure the bedroom looks really inviting. Play some great music, light candles, have drinks on hand and toys around, if that's what you both like. And remember a woman is more likely to get naked if the room feels warm!

When she arrives, lead her by the hand over to the bed where you'll have placed a pile of propped-up pillows. All the action's going to take place here with your laptop on hand. You're going to be her guide through the sex ed show. Start out with the "G-Regions" episode. It's going to fascinate and turn her on - be prepared for her to take time with each episode. It'll be worth the wait because she's soon going to be raring to start exploring.

When you've both watched samples from "Shallowing" and "Broadening" (when you activate the entire clit rather than just one part of it) tell her, "I have some homework ideas." Get the show on the road by kissing and caressing her all over her body before doing some "*Broadening.*" Sit her on top of you and tell her to slip her clit back and forward on that slippery lubed dick of yours as you stroke her nipples. When you feel her skin flush and her moans amp up, get on top of her and slowly enter her—but remember, only go an inch in. You're going to reap the benefits when she can't bear the pleasure any more and releases in an explosive orgasm that's going to feel like she's milking your dick.

Oh my, and the night's not over yet. Start to play with her vulva. Explore the wall of her vagina with your hands. Feel the bumps and creases and folds inside her—like a fingerprint, it's her own individual vagina print. Find where she's most sensitive and if she's more of a "puller," a "walker" or a "sandwich." It won't be long before she'll be panting with ecstasy as a series of new sensations in her "G Regions," unlike anything she's felt before, starts coursing through her body.

What a lesson! The good news is this is a big website. There are hours more "homework" the two of you can look forward to.

No. 14 OMGYES!

INGREDIENTS

1 OMGyes.com Season Two subscription (put in omgyes.com/101nights for your discount)

1 big bottle of lube

1 sex god-in-the-making

IMPORTANT NOTE:
This is the first time I've ever recommended a website that requires a paid subscription. I don't make any money from this, but that's how strongly I believe in what it can do for you and your sex life.

SEND HER THE TEASER!

TYPE THE LINK BELOW. CASE SENSITIVE.

101nights.com/OMGYes

MY SEX WORLD WAS ROCKED RECENTLY WHEN I came across a new experience called OMGyes.com. It does a very simple thing: asks thousands of ordinary women what feels good to them. Then it takes that information and, with the help of some incredible clips and state-of-the-art Silicon Valley graphics, teaches other women how to do those moves.

But actually, it's important for guys to get an advanced sexual education, too—and that's just what you're going to be doing this week. You're going to sign up to OMGyes.com, buy a big bottle of lube, and invite your lady to go to sex ed *with you*. OMG, YES, YOU ARE! She's going to be totally excited, because a guy who offers to attend a class to become a better lover is guaranteed to make a woman melt. Remember what I've always told you: Smart = sexy and action = attraction.

Sometimes it can be hard to "crack the code" of the female body, especially if your partner is shy about communicating. That's where OMGyes.com comes in. You'll watch women revealing their innermost sexuality secrets in a series of clips that will leave you saying, *GEE!!!!! I didn't know that.* Take the elusive "G-spot:" You've probably heard of this mind-blowing pleasure zone, but do you know how to "*Sandwich*" her G-spot, let alone "*Walk*," "*Pulsate*," or "*Pull*" it?! And do you know what "shallowing" is, perchance? It's a type of penetration I'm guessing you've never heard of; turns out that over 80% of women absolutely LOVE it.

But before you invite her to this ultimate sex education class, you're going to give yourself a sneak preview. Click on the "G-Regions" episode and you'll learn, for instance, that the mythical "G-Spot" is not a spot at all – it's a whole area. And while 48% of women have theirs on the top wall of the vagina, 16% have theirs on the bottom, while 20% of women say their G-region seems to move around!

Now check out the "*Shallowing*" episode. "Shallowing" means penetrating only an inch into

NO. 15

HEELS OVER HEAD

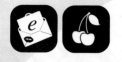

them with one of those heavenly scented softener sheets. Take a shower with a scrumptious soap and fragrant shampoo. Plan a meal (or grab some take-out) featuring your favorite foods, so that your home is filled with a mouthwatering aroma. Place a note in a spot where your guy will see it when he walks in the door:

"Go take a hot shower. Put on your robe. Then come see me in the living room."

When he joins you, he'll be impressed by the scene you've created. Candles everywhere—or better yet, a fire in the fireplace. On the floor is your finest blanket, with pillows tossed around. Tell him to make himself comfortable, propped up on pillows. Set yourself up so that you're on the floor next to him, but in the opposite direction, like those two wonderful numbers 6 and 9. Relaxed on the floor (with you wearing a sexy pair of heels you know he likes, whether barely-there strappy stilettos, spiked pumps or even thigh-grazing boots) and facing one another, you can talk and catch up on the day.

When the conversation slows, tug open his robe and admire his body. Play with his penis. Lean over and give it a kiss. Shrug your robe off, slide your leg over his head, and shift into the classic *soixante-neuf* position, the famous girl-on-top sixty-nine.

As always, he will be overwhelmed by the view. The soft light in the room creates flickering shadows over the curve of your behind, hiding then revealing the pink flower hovering over his tongue. Taste him, while he tastes you. Rock your hips as you bob your head, matching him thrust for gentle thrust.

In time, your arms may grow tired, and that's when you slowly roll onto your sides, without breaking contact. Grab a pillow and put it under your head; he'll do the same. Being in the most relaxed sexual position possible you can now take all the time you want.

Feel the heat of his face on your thighs, and the warmth of his shaft on your lips. Focus on your own pleasure. Focus on his pleasure too; remarkably, you can do both. When you get close to orgasm, back off; when you sense him getting close, slow down. Like a true gourmet, you must pace yourself. Test your erotic skills: How long can you stay balanced on the edge of ecstasy? How high can you take him?

When you finally let yourself fall into a shuddering, shattering climax, take your lover with you—how long will that blissful afterglow last? Well, certainly through dinner…and until it's time for another amazing dessert!

NO. 15 HEELS OVER HEAD

INGREDIENTS

1 fireplace, or 1 dozen candles

1 aromatic dinner at home

2 bathrobes, freshly washed

2 showers

1 pair of sexy heels

blanket and pillows

SEX COMES IN SO MANY WONDERFUL VARIETIES. There's fast sex, and freaky sex. Sex as a workout, and sex as a stress reliever. Sometimes you do it to say I love you, or You turn me on, or You're forgiven, and sometimes you're just horny.

But for sweet, lazy, totally indulgent sex—sex for the pure purpose of sensual arousal—you can't beat mutual oral sex. It's the only sex act that's called by a number, and that magical number is…

Sixty-nine.

It's not just the easiest form of sex, it's also the most delicious. He gets to taste you, and inhale you. He can feel your wetness against his lips, and slide his tongue all around your most tender parts. You get to do the same with him. And it happens at the same time, which is what makes it so hot.

What's so amazing is that you both have exquisite control over each other's pleasure. Plus it's the perfect way to communicate your own satisfaction. So it's not just your bodies that form a lovely loop. Your mutual feelings of arousal are also amplified as they pass around and around, head to tail, in an intimate form of erotic feedback. In short:

The hotter you get, the hotter he feels. And vice versa.

(That's all that's required for both of you to balance on the fine edge of orgasm—not quite crossing the line, never backing far away. Because it takes so little physical effort, you can do it for as long as you like. It ends only because you are ready for it to end.)

Prepare for an evening of gourmet indulgence. Start by washing your bathrobes, and drying

SEND HIM THE TEASER!

TYPE THE LINK BELOW. CASE SENSITIVE.

101nights.com/
HeelsOverHead

NO. 16

BEAUTIFUL SPREAD

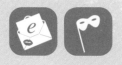

with her. Tell her how much she means to you. Tell her she's beautiful. Tell her that you fall in love with her all over again every time you see her. *Do not be embarrassed to praise her.* She longs to hear those words. If you're like most men, you probably don't say them enough. She will want to believe them.

But to completely convince her—to give her indisputable proof of how amazingly sexy she is—you've got to show her. Ask her to join you on the floor, *right in front of the mirror.* Pile some pillows on the floor for comfort, and bring the candles closer for better light. Sit down and lean against the bed for support, then ask her to sit between your legs, with her back against your chest. Make sure you can both see your reflections. Now tell her to look at herself, naked in the mirror. Rave about her body. Make her understand that this image—her, undressed, legs apart—is what you dream about. It's the most beautiful thing you know. It's the vision you have when you are making love to her, and you wanted her to see for herself just what a powerful, erotic, *perfect* sight it is. Then tell her to play with herself.

You can reach around to help her get started. If you like, you can bring out a vibrator. Run your hands over her skin. Kiss her neck. Cup her breasts while she unfolds her lips and slips her fingers between them. Soon, her fingertips will be circling faster, and she will be hypnotized by the view. And soon, because she can see *your* eyes in the mirror—because she can see the truth in them—she will come to believe you are right. She really is hot. And this is sexy, crazy-sexy, like watching another couple doing it. Like *being watched by another couple* while she masturbates. And, hello, she's feeling you get aroused behind her, too. Shift a little to one side so you can join her in self-pleasure. Stroke yourself, while she does the same, side by side. Can you time it just right? Can you watch yourselves come together? You can.

And I have a surprise for you. You'll discover it the next time you join her in the bedroom. Because you have removed much of her self-doubt, *you have made her a better lover.* And that is the real magic of the mirror.

NO.16 BEAUTIFUL SPREAD

INGREDIENTS

1 large mirror (Inexpensive models designed to hang on the back of doors work great, and you can pick one up on Amazon)

several candles

pillows or cushions

vibrator, optional

personal lubricant, optional

IT DOESN'T MATTER HOW MANY TIMES you tell her that you love her. And that she is gorgeous. And that she turns you on. Deep down inside, she still has a tiny bit of insecurity. When she looks in the mirror, she sees flaws. She can't help it. She sees Instagram models and celebrities who glow on our screens, and she can't help but feel...*ordinary*.

If only she could see herself through your eyes. Oh, wait—she *can*. You can show her exactly how hot she is. No video, no Internet, no technology required. All you need is a mirror.

Early in the day, leave a message for her. Text, phone call, or Facetime; it doesn't matter. Just tell her you have something you want to show her tonight, something hot. When evening comes around, crank up her sense of anticipation: *Chase her out of the bedroom* while you set up her surprise. I guarantee she'll be pacing on the other side of the door, like a cat in heat, waiting to get back in.

She'll expect a romantic setting in the room, and sure enough, you have candles lit and music playing. Plus there's a new addition—a good-sized mirror, propped up against the wall or the dresser. It doesn't have to be fancy or expensive, but tall enough so you can see most of yourself in the reflection. Ignore it at first. Kiss her and caress her; tug her clothes off, letting her know you want to relish every bit of her, and roll around on the bed

SEND HER THE TEASER!

TYPE THE LINK BELOW. CASE SENSITIVE.

101nights.com/
BeautifulSpread

NO. 17

I'M A SUCKER
FOR YOU

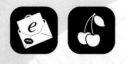

Cold beer? Cuban Cigars? Something sweet? Even if it's a sloppy meatball sub, serve it up. He's going to be elated the second he senses your attentiveness. Bring him that and more on — you guessed it — a platter. Go all out by playing his favorite music and wearing his favorite outfit. Strut into the room with your tray and say something cheesy with a sly smile, like, "Coffee, tea, or me?" Even if he's distractedly scrolling on his phone, don't be deterred.

He'll be thrilled when he sees all the treats, but the real fun hasn't even begun. Tell him to go right ahead: eat, drink, have all he wants. Then drop to your knees and work that penis like you've never worked it before. Treat it like the porn stars do with unrestrained enthusiasm. And make him believe you're feeling that growing orgasm as much as he is. Let him hear soft moans and heavy breathing. Every so often, look up at him with that half-dazed, my-god-this-feels-good expression, as if you were about to come yourself. Use every trick you know: scratch his sack, massage that sensitive spot behind his balls; slurp and nibble and take in as much as you can, for as long as you can. And remember, it's supposed to be a double-his-pleasure kind of night, so make sure he really is partaking in his other pleasures while getting pleasured by you!

The Tease you sent him a few days ago said he'd be "Top Dog" tonight, but this— well, this is top-of-the-world. It's pure, hedonistic indulgence. It's luxurious and unrestrained. It's all the best things in life.

And it's further proof that the very best thing in *his* life…is you.

NO.17 I'M A SUCKER FOR YOU

INGREDIENTS

1 perfect drink

1 perfect snack

1 perfect platter

1 perfect lover

I LIKE TO THINK THAT WE CAN ALL LEARN A little something from everyone. Porn stars, for instance. You know what makes some of them much more famous than others? It's not their beauty, or special skills, or freakish physical assets. Well, okay, for a couple of them, it is their freakish physical assets. But the popular ones, the women who actually have significant careers, all have this in common:

They look like they're enjoying it.

I mean really, really enjoying it. And not in a fake actressy way. They look like they're getting hot while doing the things that make men hot, men love this! Some of them actually believe it. And all of them want to believe it. It's a universal fantasy: I am so incredibly desirable that women get pleasure just by pleasuring me.

This week, you're going to feed him that fantasy on a platter. Literally. You're going to give him everything he loves, all his favorite indulgences at once, and he's going to believe that nothing on earth could make you happier.

What's his number one vice? Expensive brandy?

SEND HIM THE TEASER!

TYPE THE LINK BELOW. CASE SENSITIVE.

101nights.com/
ImASuckerForYou

FOR HER EYES ONLY

NO. 18

OOH-LA-LA

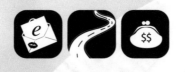

101 NIGHTS OF GREAT SEX

Let him see how excited you are as you pull them out of your shopping bag. "*Oh, honey, aren't these gorgeous! So sexy! I can't wait to try them on for you.*" Rest assured, he cannot wait to see you try them on, either. But wait he must, because this is just a tease for later in the week. Leave them out in the open, somewhere in the bedroom, so he can see them and think about them every day. Once or twice before bed, hold them up to you, over your clothes, and let him see how happy you are. Ask if he wants you to wear them, and when he says yes (or "duh!"), tell him too bad, he just has to wait a little longer. *Anticipation* means the same thing in French as in English.

On Saturday get dressed in front of him. Let him see you pull on the belt and stockings, and then hide it all away under a flattering dress. As you go about your errands, you will discover the thrill that every *jolie jeune fille* knows. When you dress well, men notice. You'll feel their eyes on you. You'll see their smiles, and sense their appreciation. You will love the attention. And you'll dig the secret thrill of traveling around town with nothing under your skirt.

This is a seduction that requires really, really, *really* good food. When it comes to cuisine, what French women sacrifice in quantity (hello, portion control), they make up for in quality. Your meal doesn't have to be French. But it should be delicious, whether you buy it from a good restaurant or make it at home. (This is a great time to try out a cooking class, by the way.) Set up a terrific meal at home. Candles, music, wine. Eat slowly, and I'll bet you both will eat less. When you get up, every click of your high heels will remind him of what you have in store.

Finally, move the action to your bedroom. Bring the candles. Set them all around you, like a halo of flickering light, so that you will be literally glowing as you unzip, unbutton, and undress for your man. Keep the lingerie on, of course. Climb on and make love the French way. *Lentement. Passionément.*

Slowly. Passionately. *Et avec du chocolat!*

NO.18 OOH-LA-LA

INGREDIENTS

1 pair of thigh-high stockings

1 garter belt

1 pair of high-heels

1 pretty dress

2 exquisite meals

many candles

THIS WEEK YOU'RE GOING TO HAVE FUN, EAT well, drive your man wild with lust…

…and lose weight.

Sounds crazy, *non*? Ah, but le*s femmes de la France* do it all the time, quite naturally, and so will you, once you see how easy and exciting it is. Your erotic play begins with some fabulous new lingerie.

French women spend a lot on lingerie, almost twenty percent of their clothing budget–the most in the Western world. Here's another question that people have been wrestling with: *How come they never seem to gain weight?* Scientists think they have an answer for that, which I don't pretend to understand. But here's Laura Corn's theory; *You can't eat much when you're wearing a garter belt.* It's a little snug around the middle. I have tested this theory, and it works! Yes, it's easier (and more comfortable) to put on thigh-highs that stay up on their own, but a garter belt is is so much more glamorous.

So go buy yourself a fantastic new garter belt and thigh-high stockings. New heels, if you want. A matching bra is a plus. But you don't need a thong. You're going to be fashionable and gloriously free under your dress. And feel reborn. *Haute* commando.

Show them to your guy when you get them home.

SEND HIM THE TEASER!

TYPE THE LINK BELOW. CASE SENSITIVE.

101nights.com/Ooh-la-la

NO. 19

DIRTY VALENTINE

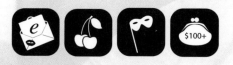

totally unexpected. Tonight you're wearing nothing but a skimpy thong with a pair of hiking boots, and perhaps a pair of plain scrunchie socks. Classic sneakers will also look super-cute if you don't have Timberlands. (You can put on your glamorous dress and high-heels afterwards.) Then just before you stroll out to see him, strap on the tool belt. He'll love the look. He'll be tickled when you tell him it's his (it's really yours!). And he'll be thrilled when he sees what you've got in it. A selection of screwdrivers? Think again.

You're packing a vibrator...a little leather flogger or paddle...bondage tape...some rope...maybe a cockring...a tube of lipstick or gloss...plus a few of your favorite bedroom accouterments...

...and a handful of Spank Ties. Have you seen these sweet things yet? They work like the little twist-ties you might use to seal bread bags, but they're made of soft, pliable rubber, about two feet long, in a luscious shade of pink. Wrap them around someone's wrists and they stay put, but are easy to escape from. They are the least threatening bondage toy ever invented. Perfect for restraining your lover on Valentine's Day.

Which is exactly what you're going to do. Make him lie down—still fully dressed—and use your Spank Ties to bind his wrists to his thighs. Set up the candles. And while you're still wearing the tool belt, slip off your thong, climb on the bed, and straddle his face. Talk dirty to him. Tell him how much you like what he's doing. Tell him to keep it up if he wants to earn a bonus present. Tell him you might even let him go free sometime tonight. If he's a good little Valentine, that is.

After several minutes, turn your attention to him. Use your happy pink ties to bind his wrists together, and his ankles, too. Unzip his pants, pull out his penis and make it hard. Make him tremble. Then straddle his hips and slip him inside you. Ride him. Rock him. Pull your vibe from the tool belt and let him watch you buzz yourself to a delicious climax, while keeping him inside you. Talk about a power drill. That image alone may be enough to push him over the top.

So are you going out for Valentine's dinner? If so, don't let him change. His slightly mussed clothes, still fragrant with the scent of sex, will make it a meal to remember. Though perhaps he'll suggest that you skip dessert. He might want to make a special after-dinner treat for you at home.

And he might want to make it with his brand new tool belt.

NO. 19 DIRTY VALENTINE

INGREDIENTS

1 traditional tool belt (they're so many surprisingly sexy ones on Amazon for less than $15!)

1 vibrator

1 bottle of personal lubricant

1 pack of batteries, if required for your vibe

3 candles

1 lighter

spank ties or rope or cuffs as an alternate

1 Valentine's Day

IMPORTANT NOTE:
This is such a GREAT IDEA that you might not want to wait for Valentine's Day! Adjust for the occasion.

SEND HIM THE TEASER!

TYPE THE LINK BELOW. CASE SENSITIVE.
101nights.com/
DirtyValentine

VALENTINE'S DAY IS NOT A PERFECT HOLIDAY. Oh, it's great, and it certainly has lots of potential every year. But for guys, V-Day represents a *hu-uu-uge* amount of pressure, with endless opportunities for getting it wrong. It can be breathtakingly expensive. (And that's if your guy doesn't collapse from decision-making paralysis and end up doing nothing, while cursing Cupid under his breath.)

Here's something else that can go wrong on Valentine's. Some couples never get around to physical intimacy! That's because the sex comes last, if it comes at all. By the end of the day they are too stuffed with fancy food, too buzzed with wine, and too stressed from the pressure of saying "I love you *this much*" to actually get down to the act of love. It's the Wedding Day Syndrome, repeated every year.

The solution is obvious. Get dirty early! And buy him something you'll both love. Something perfectly practical, yet romantic. Something simultaneously useful and hot. Get him a tool belt.

Tease him in the days leading up to Valentine's Day. Tell him often how you found the best gift for him, and that he's going to love it. Try not to laugh too loud when you see him squirm and sweat as he second-guesses his own gift for you. He may run back to the store two or three times, upgrading his present, uncertain of his own romantic judgment. Men are hilarious like that, no?

A half-hour before it's time for dinner, sneak away to put on your special Valentine's outfit. But this isn't your standard lacy lingerie. No, it's something

FOR **HIS EYES** ONLY

NO. **20**

ONE HOT DROP

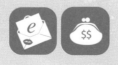

101 NIGHTS OF GREAT SEX

will grab your girl's attention. Early in the week, send her the Tease. Wait a day, then shoot her a text that says, "Up for a sex date this weekend?" Let her know which night you're thinking. She'll be more than excited to accept! When the weekend arrives, spring your surprise. Bring her to the bedroom, which is glowing by the light of a dozen candles, including your new massage candle. *"One of these candles is special,"* you tell her. *"You'll get a nice treat if you can figure out which one."*

It's okay to give her some hints. But you don't have to say too much. Forget waxing poetic; what you've got in store will speak volumes. Because the real secret isn't finding the candle, it's what comes next. Spread a couple of big towels on the bed, and ask her to sit down. Tell her to stick out her arm. Gently grasp her wrist with one hand, and pick up your massage candle with the other. Hold it several inches over her forearm, and then—slowly, dramatically—pour a few drops onto her skin.

Did her eyes pop? I'll bet they did. It's a startling thing to witness. It requires much trust, because she instinctively fears the flame and the sting. But the drops don't hurt. They feel *good*. Especially when you rub the waxy lotion into her skin, massaging her wrist and working out the tension in her hand and fingers.

Now that she's comfortable with the candle, ask her to undress and lie down on her stomach. Here comes the best part. Dribble a few drops of the luscious melted wax and spread it across her back. Let the heat soak in while you massage it into her skin. *Wow*.

Knead the tension out of her neck and shoulders. As the candle burns down, pour out more hot drops. Polish her skin. Work the kinks out of her back, then move down to her thighs and bottom. Take your time; the massage candle can burn for a long time. And in the end, it's not really gone. You've just transferred all of its heat into *her*. And what do suppose she is going to do with all that fire?

I think she's going to light your wick.

NO.20 ONE HOT DROP

INGREDIENTS

1 low-temperature massage candle (like the JimmyJane Afterglow Body Wax Massage Candle, at Amazon.com. You can also watch how to play with hot wax on Youtube.)

12 or more regular candles (to set the mood)

large bath towels

SEND HER THE TEASER!

TYPE THE LINK BELOW. CASE SENSITIVE.

101nights.com/
OneHotDrop

IT SOUNDED SO KINKY. It looked so sensual in the movies. I couldn't wait to try it. And when I did— OW! Ouch ouch ouch OUCH! *Damn*, that hurt. This is supposed to be sexy?!

Turns out I was an idiot. I didn't do it right the first time. But *you* will. And your partner will learn what I finally did—that there is some extraordinary pleasure to be found in playing with hot wax.

Lots of erotic books and movies feature a scene where a man holds a burning candle and lets melted wax slowly drip onto the skin of his lover. Hot, slippery goo; a hint of S&M? Wow. Yes. That makes me tingle. And I'm not the only woman turned on by those scenes. I wrote about it in my blog, and got rave responses from hundreds of women, who all thought it was an awesome fantasy. But reality turned out to be trickier than I had imagined. That's because regular candle wax melts at way too high a temperature. Those drops burn, baby! And when they cool, they stick to your body hairs like bubble gum. My first attempt was a complete mess. And did I mention the *ouch*?

But there are candles specially made to burn at low temperatures. The melted wax is deliciously warm to the touch, but not too hot. My favorite kind is the Afterglow Massage Candle by JimmyJane, created specifically for sex play. The wax is not just body-friendly, it actually melts into a natural massage oil.

As always, you should start with something that

FOR HER EYES ONLY

NO. 21

BOND GIRL

101 NIGHTS OF GREAT SEX

Sure, you had his attention the moment he started getting aroused, but now he's just fascinated. It's flattering, this extra penile attention. It's wickedly interesting, this tight elastic sensation. And when you start tugging on the hair bands, pulling his shaft back and forth, up and down, bumping the crown against your cheeks and your lips, well, it's just unbelievably hot. The extra squeeze from your homemade penis ring keeps him nice and hard, and ready for fun.

Take your time. Go slow. Slide the elastic bands up and down. Pull them away from his skin—just a tiny fraction of an inch, just barely off the surface, just enough to make his eyes go wide and then let him snap back into place. And again, a little harder. Keep the tip in your mouth, sucking just hard enough to curl his toes, but not so hard that he pops before you're done with him. Mmmm, that's a delicate balance there, but I know you can do it.

Finally, using lips and teeth only—start to remove the stretchy ties. Suck, and then tug. Pull one off, then suck some more. Make him wait! You are the goddess of his penis, and you have the skill to delay his orgasm until the last tie is off, and in your mouth.

NO. 21 BOND GIRL

INGREDIENTS

3-4 ponytail holders (extra points if they're cute)

HERE'S SOMETHING THEY DIDN'T TEACH YOU in Sex Ed class: How to keep your hair out of the way when you're going down on a man. Yet every woman eventually figures it out. Hair Ties = Easier Ponytails = Better Blowjobs.

This seduction is short and sweet yet yields big results. Start by sending your man the Tease, so you both can get ready for a game of bonding! Some of the best ideas are really simple—and come out of good, old common sense. Who knew wearing a ponytail holder (or three) could catalyze a night of hot sex?! When you're ready to go, put your hair up in not one but several stretchy hair ties and let the games begin. Get him all good and hard, then…pull one of the elastic ties out of your hair and slide it down over his shaft. Get a second one, pull it wide open, and slip it on, too, a couple of inches away from the first.

SEND HIM THE TEASER!

TYPE THE LINK BELOW. CASE SENSITIVE.

101nights.com/BondGirl

FOR **HIS EYES** ONLY

NO. 22

FIFTY SHADES
OF PLEASURE

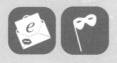

feel of her cheeks in your palms, and you controlling her. If she tries to squirm or move away, don't let her.

Spanking is as much about power play as it is about sensation. Just knowing that you are in charge is enough to excite her from head to toe. Whisper "Don't move," and you've got her: she'll be dying to kiss you, touch you, and show you how much she wants you. But you've commanded her not to. That's the first step.

I want you to tell her, "You've been a bad girl." Whether she has or not, by this point, she'll want to be "bad." It's all part of a ritual, a process, and the lead-up is often the most arousing part. Ask her why she's been naughty and if she needs to be punished. Get her to admit that she wants to be spanked.

Get comfortable. Now comes one of the most important moments: the first smack. Do not hit her as hard as you can. Do not let out all your pent-up lust on this first go. Tap her ass to start. One cheek, then the next. See how she reacts. Then do it a little harder. There's a build-up. Make sure you hear that gratifying smack! (Tip: It's often in the flick of the wrist.) Get a rhythm going and observe what she does. If you're not sure, ask her if she wants it harder or run your finger between her legs to see how wet she is. Hold her down with the nonspanking hand in the small of her back. Tell her how hard spanking her is making you. Listen to the sound your hand makes against her skin, and hear her breathing change as she gets more turned on.

The "sweet spot" is generally the middle of her ass, where both cheeks meet, and the backs of her upper thighs are fun too. You'll soon see how excited she is, as well as the visible marks of your handiwork.

I want you to stop just when you're both going into overdrive. Lightly stroke her bottom with your hand, or bring her up for a kiss before you return to the spanking. Tease her by holding off from giving her what she really wants, until neither of you can stand to wait any longer.

When you're done spanking, anything goes.

NO.22 FIFTY SHADES OF PLEASURE

INGREDIENTS

your imagination

patience

her bare bottom

1 flogger (optional)

YOU LOVE HER, AND WANT TO MAKE HER HAPPY.
But sometimes, you can't help but picture what she'd look like draped over your knee, naked, as she waits for you to dish out her "punishment." Here's a secret: She probably dreams about the same thing, but asking to be spanked isn't always easy, even though it's far less taboo than it used to be. Which is exactly why you should take her over your knee and turn her bottom red!

But before you do, send her the Tease. That way, she'll know something exciting is happening this week. Pick the right time for your sex date and tell her when to meet you in the bedroom. Then it's bottoms up!

One of women's most erogenous zones is on their bottoms; getting spanked stimulates her clitoris, which, coupled with the feeling of "giving herself over" to you, physically and figuratively, can make her go wild. If she's already aroused, all the better. Start by showing some major appreciation for her ass; you don't just want to spank it, but stroke it, squeeze it, fondle it, kiss it, caress it, until all she wants is for you to keep going.

Soon it will be time to drape her over your knee. But before you do, blindfold her and restrain her hands behind her back. If she has long hair, watch it fall to the ground. Whatever the length, give it a little tug to remind her she's fully succumbing. When the moment is right, bring your hands to her ass and just hold them there. Get used to the

SEND HER THE TEASER!

TYPE THE LINK BELOW. CASE SENSITIVE.

101nights.com/
FiftyShadesOfPleasure

NO. 23

BAD TO
THE BONER

This accomplishes two key things: It gets her aroused, all week long. And it gives her a chance to put on her best panties. Hey, we want to look good when we're getting ravished. That's part of the fantasy, too.

On the night when you finally get to be really bad, you need to be really good first. Text her: *You don't need to deal with a thing tonight. I've got you.* That also means eliminating the things that distract her: bring home a nice dinner, take care of the kids, put clean sheets on the bed. (One of my girlfriends says that the sexiest thing in the world is the sound of a man cleaning up the kitchen. I don't think she's kidding.) Give her a chance to relax in a hot bath, and let voicemail do its job for the rest of the night.

Tell her to call you when she's ready to get out of the tub (that's right, tonight you're not asking, you're telling). You'll be waiting with a warm towel to wrap her up. Have her robe standing by. Now it's time to turn off the sweetness. Be direct. Grab her as she's putting on her robe; push her up against the wall. (Then again, she might not have a chance to even put it on and that's more than fine.) Then carry her over to the bed. Lie her down, so you can fully take over. Start with your tongue, but don't make her come, not just yet. Women appreciate the incredible difference between the feel of your mouth and the feel of your penis, so give her some of both. Go down on her for a few minutes, then change. Pump her slow and steady, then switch back to using your tongue. A-a-a-annnd repeat.

No one's keeping score here. But you want a number, don't you? Guys always want a number. So, six. Six times back and forth. At least.

Then kick it up a notch. Climb on top and grab her wrists, pinning them to the pillow above her head. A simple move, sure, but right now it's like throwing gasoline on a fire. Keep feeding her fantasy by being totally dominant: pull her across the sheets, roll her over, let her feel your weight and your strength. Don't worry about being fair, not tonight. She's getting exactly what she wants because you're taking what you want.

NO. 23 BAD TO THE BONER

INGREDIENTS

1 badass motherfucka

1 night with no distractions
(Take care of kids, dinner,
bath, clean sheets)

*"They are the men of our dreams. The word
'bad' doesn't even begin to describe their
wicked ways. With just a look, they can
jump-start our deepest desires."*

I Love Bad Boys
LORI FOSTER, JANELLE DENISON, DONNA KAUFFMAN

She wants a bad boy. You know she does. And
since the publication of the best-selling book *Fifty
Shades of Grey*, she wants one even more (yes, even
in the age of #MeToo).

And it's not just her. Turns out it's the number
one fantasy among women; that wicked guy who
just takes her. Tosses her on the bed, rips off her
panties, does her hard. Then does her again. Not
exactly politically correct—but it's hot.

But, as with so many great fantasies, there are a
few problems with turning it into reality. For one
thing, no woman in her right mind wants a bad
boy all the time. They're bad! And then there's the
problem of scheduling. All that raw, immediate,
butt-slapping sex sounds great in theory, but real
life has kids and jobs and housework. Not to
mention PMS.

So here's the solution. Plan your spontaneous sex.
Pick a time when you know she won't be wiped
out from work. Warm her up early in the week
with the Bad To The Boner Teaser.

SEND HER
THE TEASER!

TYPE THE LINK BELOW. CASE SENSITIVE.

101nights.com/
BadToTheBoner

NO. 24

MAN HANDLER

again with your hand. This may sound silly, but get a fresh manicure before you show off your new handjob skills. If he's got a favorite shade (pale pink and flaming red tend to be favorites), go for it. The site of your gorgeous, gleaming hands on him will pump up the experience, pun intended.

If you're going to go up against a master at the peak of his game, then you're also going to need to learn a few pro tricks yourself. Fortunately, there's a delightful YouTube video featuring a group of women who uses a life-sized plastic models to show you exactly how it's done. These demonstrations are amazing! To quote one of the comments, "If every woman took this class in school, the world would be a better place." Haha! These lovely ladies show you more than twenty specialized techniques for using your hands to get a guy off, but you only need to learn a few.

1) **Lock and Load:** Wrap both your hands around his shaft and lock your fingers together. Then, quickly slide your hands up and down and twist them from side to side—great when it's time for the big finish.

2) **Milking The Bull:** Alternate using each of your hands to pull up on his penis, so that as soon as one hand gets to the tip, the other starts, creating one continuous motion—like he's pulling out of a never-ending vagina.

3) **The Slippy Grippy** (it's even fun just to say out-loud!): Use your nonperforming hand to grip the base of the penis. This stabilizes it and allows your stronger hand to grab onto the end with as much force and strength as you like

Go forth, young student. Learn the handjob. Become the handjob. Later this week, a few hours before you plan to debut your new skills, hand your man a big new bottle of Astroglide or other slick sex lubricant. Smile and say, "Bring this to bed tonight. I wouldn't want you to get hurt."

Now *there's* a challenge no guy will turn down.

no. 24 MAN HANDLER

INGREDIENTS

1 *big* bottle of Astroglide or other sex lubricant.

2 strong hands

1 Internet connection

1 visit to Youtube (search for the following video: Handjob for a man, How-to, Masterclass, Tutorial. Demonstration on a Toy)

FOR COUPLES WHO TRULY WANT TO LEARN how to light their sheets on fire, the Internet is something close to a miracle. And no, I'm not talking about the porn that comes oozing out of your screen every time you turn around. (Holy St. Jenna, most of it is so *lame*! Who knew sex could look so cheap?!)

What makes the Internet so inspiring for aspiring lovers is the instructional videos. While our dependency on technology can sometimes make great sex harder to achieve (short attention spans! The urge to check Instagram!), there's a lot to appreciate about in this wonderful age of instant techno-sex. Why not use it to master more sexual techniques? They're right at your fingertips.

This week you're going to study the art of manual stimulation or, as it is classically and lovingly referred to, the handjob. Many women mistakenly assume the handjob is easy; a tug, a jiggle, then get out the Kleenex. But consider this—the guy you are trying to impress has been playing this game virtually every day of his pubescent life. He is Tom Brady; he is Tiger Woods—a man who has known for years the power and strength of the hand.

While we might not have quite as much practice with his penis, we do have a couple advantages. Feminine wiles and the refreshing unfamiliarity of a new hand. You can seduce your man all over

SEND HIM
THE TEASER!

TYPE THE LINK BELOW. CASE SENSITIVE.

101nights.com/
ManHandler

FOR HER EYES ONLY

NO. 25

BEST.ONE.EVER.

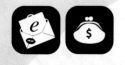

101 NIGHTS OF GREAT SEX

And nothing proves this point more than taking a photo right after you have sex. A well-fucked woman is a beautiful thing to see!

So this week you're going to snap a picture of you and your honey right after making love. The GLOW (and visible connection between you and your partner) is UNMISTAKABLE.

By capturing a photo in those precious moments, the ephemeral becomes eternal. You can't put a price on love, but you can capture it!

And now I'm going to show you how to take the ultimate post-sex selfie.

First, you want to think about how you're going to take the picture before you and your honey have sex, and that's the fun part. Muse on the kind of sex you want to have. What makes you feel the glowy-est after? Slow and soft love-making with lots of kissing? Or wild and crazy, down-and-dirty sex? Ask yourself if you feel hottest when you're on top, taking charge? With his head buried between your legs? Do you like hazy, lazy morning sex? A naughty afternoon delight? Or late at night, deep in the dark? You know what gives you that GLOW!

Set up the scene in your mind beforehand. What will you be wearing? (Something lacy? Next to nothing?!) Which angle do you like best? (Selfies tend to be most flattering when taken from slightly above.) What kind of lighting do you prefer? (Natural light during twilight, also known as the magic hour, is gorgeous.) The point is to envision it in your mind – then start snapping away within five minutes of having sex. I put on lipstick and combed my hair, but that's it! Finally, decide if you want to let your man know beforehand.

Whether you take the photo in bed, tangled in the sheets, or sitting on a chair together (I sat on Jeff's lap for mine), just have fun with your #justmadelove photo. You can even scan Instagram for ideas. Look at photos of other couples and see if you can notice *that glow*. I know I can tell! Check out A-Rod and Jennifer Lopez's Instagram accounts. Those two are having lots of great SEX!

Speaking of *that* glow, you'll see it right away. You'll see the love. The passion. The intimacy. The spark.

Once you've selected your favorite photo, get it printed and nicely framed. Finally, hang it up on your bedroom wall or put it on your nightstand, so every time you walk into your room, you'll be reminded how important physical intimacy is. It's one of the most meaningful photos the two of you will ever take, and I recommend taking one every year.

The right picture *is* worth a thousand words, but it's also worth *a thousand orgasms!*

INGREDIENTS

1 camera or smartphone

1 ready and willing partner

THEY SAY A PICTURE IS WORTH A THOUSAND words, and I couldn't agree more. A picture is also worth a *book deal* with the biggest publisher in the world!

It happened over 15 years ago and all started with a dry spell. Over two months had passed since I'd had sex with my longtime partner, Jeff. Needless to say, I was feeling down; my smile and spark had completely disappeared. I didn't just notice this when I looked in the mirror; *there was visible proof in the photos we were taking*.

That's when I had an epiphany! No sex = No glow. I instantly flipped the switch and as soon as we had sex, I felt better. For the next month, we had record amounts of sex, and I took a whole lot of photos, documenting my reawakening.

My little experiment inspired an idea. I wanted to take it on the road and find out if other couples could see the difference, too. I tested this theory out on 38 couples, who took "before" photos, during their dry spell, and then captured themselves 30 days later, after a lot of sex. Boy, was I right! Not only did we look better, we looked years younger!

I brought these results to New York, and presented the idea to the pubishing house HarperCollins, along with the concept of my book *The Great American Sex Diet*. When I showed everyone the photos they were *blown away*! Before I knew it, the team was consulting with billionaire Rupert Murdoch (owner of HarperCollins) who couldn't wait to offer me a book deal. Clearly, I was onto something BIG.

I'm not telling you this to brag but to prove a potentially life-changing point: You can see a HUGE visible difference in yourself *and* in your relationship when your sex life is flourishing.

SEND HIM THE TEASER!

TYPE THE LINK BELOW. CASE SENSITIVE.

101nights.com/
BestOneEver

NO. 26

DINNER PARTY

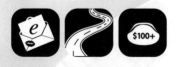

"off-limits" ideas you've yet to explore. Or those things you used to do in the past that you haven't for way too long. Or perhaps best of all, something he's mentioned he would love but has never actually happened. This menu is made for them!

Below are some of my own personal menu choices that bring new meaning to the term *hot* dish. Let them get your taste buds tingling and add in some of your own!

Appetizers
- I take my panties off and spread my legs the whole way home.
- Watch me play with myself using something in the glove box.*
- I stroke you all the way home.
- Kiss me (and maybe pull my hair and nibble my ears) at every red light.
- I press my naked breasts up against the window (or up against you).
- Two words: Road head.

Remember to "accidentally" leave a vibrator there.

Entrées
- I get on all fours and deep-throat you.
- Film me with your phone while I'm going down on you.
- Rip off my dress and throw me on the bed – or floor.
- Watch me do a striptease to the song of your choice.
- Do me anywhere and everywhere in the house, in any position you want (reverse cowgirl included).
- Once we go to sleep, you have permission to wake me up anytime and do *anything* you want.

Side Dishes
- I whisper nasty things in your ear.
- Put a leash around my neck and tell me what to do.
- Give me a hickey wherever you want.
- I'll put on any outfit you want.
- I sit on your face.
- I give extra attention to your pulsing, hard penis.

Dessert
- I make your favorite snack and serve it to you in bed. Maybe with a bottle of wine.
- You get a long massage.
- No talking, no cuddling, just straight-up hot sex.
- I sleep naked all night.
- Make me the dessert with the help of some whipped cream.
- Round two! Or three!

Throughout your meal, he's going to find himself pondering the eight items he wants most. Use this time to indulge your inner flirt. Let the strap of your dress fall off your shoulder to reveal a little more cleavage. "Accidentally" brush your hand against his crotch as you get up to go to the ladies' room. Turn back around to give him a sly smile while you strut away. Make him feel like he's the only person in the place when you walk back by gazing at him with wanting eyes. Don't be surprised if he can't take his hands and eyes off you as you discuss the menu options throughout the evening. He may want a little more information on certain items, which you'll assuredly offer up and if you're feeling especially generous (or particularly horny), you may let him spring for nine instead of eight. The only rule is to flirt, tease and enjoy the anticipation.

At the end of dinner, which might come quicker than most meals, he's going to hand your menu back with his final choices circled. By now, a whole new thrill has kicked in. Pay the bill, walk outside and take a look at the winning dishes: It's time to bring this dinner to a whole new level. Who's the *Top Chef* now? Next time, he's going to want to wine you, dine you and yes, sixty-nine you. It's one thing to serve dinner and it's another entirely to serve your man. You'd be amazed the response you get from a man once he knows you've put in a little effort for him. Whether they admit it or not, men *love* attention. They *need* validation and often this comes in the form of sex. By taking initiative and going into dinner with an open mind (and perhaps open legs), you've created a fun-filled night of mind-blowing sex, not to mention one with an equally electrifying lead-up.

Don't be surprised if he makes a reservation for the same restaurant, and that same back banquette, next week!

INGREDIENTS

1 sheet of A4 paper

Colored pens or printer ink

1 up-for-anything attitude

THE DINNER DATE IS ONE OF THE MAINSTAYS of any relationship and while it's almost always fun to go to your favorite restaurant, after a while you know *exactly* what to expect. You discuss which appetizers to share (calamari again?), mull over springing for that full bottle of wine and each talk about your day. Not this time! Tonight you're going to host a very different kind of dinner party—and trust, by the end of the evening you will definitely have earned your title as *hostess with the mostest*. We all know nothing keeps the spark in a relationship alive like the element of surprise, but you're not one to settle for the minimum. How about reigniting a full-fledged flame? Enter the Back Banquette.

Here's how it works: start by planning ahead. Mid-week, send him a text saying, *We're going out to dinner Saturday night. Get ready for a special meal and then some.*

Make reservations at one of your favorite dinner restaurants, one with deliciously dark lighting and an atmosphere that sets the mood. Be sure to book the sexy back booth; a little privacy will come in handy. Extra points if it's roomy enough for you to sit next to each other—you'll radiate more heat if you're seductively close-by. When the night comes, you're going to slink into that banquette wearing your hottest dress, sharpest stilettos and most importantly, an air of tantalizing confidence and say to him, "Baby, I hope you're hungry. Once you order from the menu, I've got a second menu here designed just for you."

His interest will be piqued. While he might try to press you for more details, tell him he has to wait and see. This is a playful game and as long as he knows it's all in good fun, dinner is foreplay for the *other* courses. Once he's ordered his prime rib and you've both settled into your cocktails, present him with your own gorgeous menu, either handwritten or printed-out, outlining the irresistible à la carte options you've got planned for him later.

Pass him an inky pen (a Bic ballpoint just isn't sexy) and tell him he can make eight choices from your sizzling-hot menu:

- **Two Appetizers** (*racy foreplay for the car ride home*)
- **Two Entrées** (*more substantial fare for when you're back at home*)
- **Two Side Dishes** (*sexual add-ons to embellish your main course*)
- **Two Desserts** (*post-climax treats*)

Remember to be clever here. This night is for him, but it's wise to put items on the menu you've always fantasized about but have never gotten around to trying. That's the beauty of the Back Booth; it inspires you to play with some sexy, often

SEND HIM THE TEASER!

TYPE THE LINK BELOW. CASE SENSITIVE.

101nights.com/
DinnerParty

NO. **27**

SPLASH
OF SEXY

Yes, I mean still dressed in your undies. No, he will not think it's strange. He will think it's way hot, because, let's face it, it is. Warm water, slippery skin, wet fabric — he'll think he woke up in the uncensored version of Girls Gone Wild. Except sober.

Now work it like you're in a wet t-shirt contest with a million-dollar prize. Survivor: Spring Break. Lather up, letting your soapy fingers slide all over the nearly transparent fabric. Rub your slick body against him. It doesn't seem like much, but that one extra layer makes it so very, very naughty. Plus there's that whole extra rush that comes from knowing you were so turned on that you couldn't even stop to take off your clothes. Or so he thinks. Bonus fun: use one of those detachable massage shower-heads. Double bonus fun: use a waterproof vibrator.

And don't worry about running out of hot water. You two can make your own steam.

NO.27 SPLASH OF SEXY

INGREDIENTS

1 tight white t-shirt

1 pair of white cotton panties

1 hot shower

Optional: 1 Waterproof Vibrator

I INTERVIEWED MORE THAN 1,000 MEN AND asked them to tell me about their most memorable sexual experiences. And almost every single one had something in common; they started spontaneously.

Spontaneity rocks. But do you know what can make it even better? A little bit of planning. Hey, don't tell me that it doesn't make sense. We're talking about great sex here. Sometimes logic has nothing to do with it.

First, plan your spontaneous sex for a morning when your guy is not on a tight schedule. Deadlines and erections don't mix. Second, plan your outfit. I personally think you can't go wrong with a tight white t-shirt and white cotton panties and I'm willing to bet he agrees. Last, wait for him to climb into the shower and then — surprise! — spontaneously join him.

SEND HIM THE TEASER!

TYPE THE LINK BELOW. CASE SENSITIVE.

101nights.com/
SplashOfSexy

NO. 28

SEX SPA

she reminds you of that, just let her know it'll be worth her while to shake up her routine.) That evening, get things ready by getting a chair and putting it in the middle of the bathroom. Spread the towels everywhere, across the chair and floor. Then invite her into the bathroom, leading her into the already-running shower. Finally, get undressed and join her in there, as you hand her a gift-wrapped present.

It's a new bottle of shampoo, deliciously scented. Her mood will shift from shocked—*he brought me a giftwrapped package in the shower!*—to surprised—*hey, he bought me a gift*—and finally to totally seduced, after you offer to wash her hair. Let me tell you, this is one truly erotic sensation for a woman. It's luxurious, it's sensual, it's hot, and she's probably going to want to do you right then and there—but be patient. I promise, it'll be worth the wait.

Now lather. Rinse. Repeat. And then lead her out of the shower into the hot, steamy bathroom. Write a message on the mirror with your finger: "I Want You." Then take her. Dripping wet. Soaked through. Slick and steamy and drenched with water. Don't dry off; the towels are there only for cleanup and for cushioning. Do it on the chair and on the counter. Do it in the tub and on the floor. Do it until the whole room is splattered and wet. And keep doing it until...

...well, until you both need to jump in the shower again.

NO. 28 SEX SPA

INGREDIENTS

Lots of towels, fresh out of the dryer

1 sturdy chair

1 shower

1 finger-written note on the bathroom mirror

1 bottle of shampoo, nicely gift-wrapped (Check out Strawberry Clearly Glossing shampoo at "The Body Shop")

I LOVE WET SEX. Sex in the pool, sex in the shower, sex in a hot tub. And it's not just me. Every woman I know says she enjoys it more when there's water involved. Partly that's because we know we look good, all glistening and moist, like some beer commercial come to life. And sure, the whole slip-n-slide element makes it fun.

But mostly it's because we really, really like to be clean and fresh when we're about to start bumping our tingly parts against yours. And you know what? We really like it when *you're* shiny and well-scrubbed, too. Clean enough to eat off of.

But this encounter goes beyond just wet. It's *sloppy*, and that's why you need to make sure you're stocked up on great big bath towels this week. Ask her which night she's planning on washing her hair. She'll probably ask why and you'll respond casually, *"I'm prepping seduction #55."* Anticipation in place! I bet she'll giggle, *"Tonight!"* (Even if she usually washes her hair in the morning. And if

SEND HER THE TEASER!

TYPE THE LINK BELOW. CASE SENSITIVE.

101nights.com/SexSpa

FOR **HIS EYES** ONLY

NO. **29**

CHILL
TO THRILL

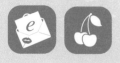

101 NIGHTS OF GREAT SEX

At dinner, look at her pointedly, keeping your cool. The anticipation is *killing* her. Go about your evening as usual, but catch her eye occasionally and wink. She likes that you have a secret.

When dessert time nears, walk behind her and whisper, *Don't forget, dessert reservations at 8:30!* Once she's gone, lay napkins and your ice cream bars on a plate or tray. Stand tall, shoulders back. You are cool and your lady is waiting.

Walk confidently into the room, telling her to keep her eyes closed. Ask if she's ready for dessert. Stay in character! She might giggle or ask what you're doing. She's naked underneath her robe, blinded, and nervous about what might happen. Good! She's nervous with anticipation, and that's *exactly* what you want.

With her eyes still closed, unwrap the bar. Make a lot of noise with the wrapper. Let her hear it crinkle. Stand very close so she can feel your heat. Trace the skin of her neck, shoulders, and nipples through the fabric of her robe with your fingers. Untie the front; let it drop to the floor. *Shivers...*

Watch her face. Listen to her breathing. Move the bar close to her body. Trace the same path, but this time drag the tip of the treat along her skin. Be prepared for her to gasp, jump, and squirm while you take your time.

Use your voice to send shivers down her spine: *Your skin is so soft...your nipples get so hard when I touch them...you look so sexy with your eyes closed...*Wield the stick like a paintbrush. Write your name across her body. The bar is melting now, leaving sweet drips. *Slowly*, erase each drop with your tongue.

By now she knows what you're holding, and you're both excited. It's time to make good on your promise of dessert. Stand in front of her, touch the treat's tip to her lips, and pull back. Tease her with it. *Show me your tongue...*let her have a lick. Keep the treat in front of her mouth, just out of reach. Watch as she searches, allowing her a lick. Pull it away and take a few bites. *So good. I bet you'd like a bite, wouldn't you?*

Walk around her as if you're contemplating what you'll do. Stop directly in front of her. *Open your eyes.* Give her the last bite, kiss the taste from her lips and say, *Take off my clothes.* You've been direct, confident and commanding. You've made her feel excited, vulnerable, and sexy. Enjoy the view as she undresses you.

It's sex-on-a-stick time.

INGREDIENTS

Ice cream bars or other frozen treats on a stick

a small plate

a big attitude

FAMED ICE CREAM MAKER HÄAGEN-DAZS has long emphasized the sensual delights of its products by creating ads that show lovers licking ice cream from their partners' bodies. Tonight, you're going to utilize the sexual power of ice cream…and, trust me, this is one time she won't care about the calories!

Tonight's encounter is all about order and control. As much as women want to share responsibilities, there's a little part of us that really likes it when you take charge. When your passion and confidence combines—*boom!* We forget we ever wanted equality in the first place.

Plant the seed of tonight's seduction. Tell her you've got a surprise and you want her to play along. When she agrees, look her confidently in the eye and say, *I'll be taking care of dessert tonight.* Let her think you're being a typical, predictable guy planning to let her have *you* for dessert. She'll think she's got you all figured out.

Send her the Teaser first thing in the morning and make sure she reads it. Then around noon, send this text with your command: *Dessert will be served in the bedroom tonight at 8:30 PM sharp. You should be standing in the middle of the floor, naked under your robe, with your eyes closed. Don't be late.* Be direct, confident. She'll be completely turned on by the thought of waiting for you.

Pick up a box of ice cream bars. Dove Bars are perfect: yummy chocolate (the closest thing to sex for many of us), smooth vanilla ice cream, and an easy-to-grip stick. Choose a non-dairy version if you've noticed she's on an almond milk kick lately. Either way, you'll appreciate the grip later; trust me. Stash them in the freezer.

SEND HER THE TEASER!

TYPE THE LINK BELOW. CASE SENSITIVE.

101nights.com/ ChillToThrill

NO. 30

ESCAPE ROOM

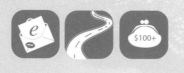

out the door. What?! Holy Cow! A secret message in my favorite magazine? She'll fly through the pages until she comes to your note which is taped inside: "HEY, STELLA, THIS IS IT! There's a gift hidden in one of the bedrooms. Find it, and follow the instructions."

Wouldn't you just love to see her tearing through the house looking for her present? This is where your credit card starts to warm up, because the gift has to be pretty nice—a sexy teddy or lacy camisole. Laura Corn Shopping Tip for Men: A slinky robe is easy to fit, since they only come in small, medium and large. (They're also easy to return. Just in case.) If lingerie shops make you feel a little uneasy, get something gorgeous from VictoriasSecret.com.

Your package must be gift-wrapped, of course. When she finally spots it, the first thing she'll see is a big note that says:

> "DO NOT OPEN! Bring this to the Sheraton on Broadway at 6 p.m. and ask for Woody Johnson. Your next big surprise is waiting there."

Ohhh, yes. Yes, yes, yes, she's getting more excited now. She's got just enough time to get dressed and call all her girlfriends to tell them how cool you are. Once you get to the hotel room, send her a few texts—enticing her as she gets ready.

The hotel clerk will direct her to your room. (Woody Johnson!? I wonder if he'll be able to keep a straight face.) The clerk will also call to let you know she's on the way, so you can light the candles, turn up the music, and pop the cork. Now, can you just imagine what she's got for you in return?

Woody, you haven't got a clue!

NO.30 ESCAPE ROOM

INGREDIENTS

1 handwritten note "taped inside" a magazine (yes, she still reads them at the beauty salon!)

1 e-mail or text message

1 sexy teddy or robe

1 hotel room

ALL TREASURE HUNTS REQUIRE some advance work. Maybe that's why women love them so much. There's great presentation, plus a great present at the end of it all.

This little rendezvous is more of a pleasure hunt, of course. And the coolest thing about it is that you get a lot of bang for the buck. It's extremely impressive, and it looks like you worked really hard. But, in fact, it's pretty easy: a couple of phone calls, a little online shopping, a ding on the credit card, and you're golden. She'll get a sexy adventure she'll be telling her friends about for years. And you're set for an adventure in great sex.

Your first step is to let her know that something's up. Spontaneity is great, but a girl's gotta prepare, you know? So early in the week, send her a text: "I know what you like. And you're gonna get it this Saturday. Don't make any plans after 4p.m." (Didn't I say I'd make this easy?)

Saturday afternoon, hand her her favorite magazine (anything about celebrities will do) and tell her, "Look inside. There's a secret message waiting for you." Now give her a kiss and walk

SEND HER THE TEASER!

TYPE THE LINK BELOW. CASE SENSITIVE.

101nights.com/
EscapeRoom

NO. 31

#LOVESEXMUSIC

Wow you just hit it out of the park. She's feeling hot & beautiful.

Just remember to save every song she sends you to your growing playlist (if you're using songs from mine, save her songs and then create an original list that combines them both).

Every few hours, send another song. Go literal and let the lyrics speak for you. From the classic ("Let's Get It On" by Marvin Gaye) to the campy ("Take My Breath Away" by Berlin) to the sex-crazed (hello, "Pony" by Ginuwine), every choice sends a message designed to make her feel adored, feel appreciated, and feel just how badly you want her.

By the time the evening of your date rolls around, not only have you reminded her of the deep connection you share, which is always a major turn-on for women, you've created an original playlist together, the perfect soundtrack for your night. Put it on without saying anything and draw her close to you, that knowing glint in her eyes. Maybe you'll dance to the first couple of jams or maybe you'll get right down to it.

This seduction is as mentally engaging as it is exciting: For the last several days, you've been speaking in your own private language no one else in the world can understand. What's sexier than that? Talk about harmony! By the time you're deep inside her, you might want to listen to some of the hottest sounds of all: the two of you in the throes of passion – and all the moans, grunts, exclamations and hopefully dirty talk that comes with it.

It'll be music to her ears.

POTENTIAL PLAYLIST OPTIONS, JUST TO START:

"Feel like Makin' Love" by Roberta Flack
"Adorn" by Miguel
"Pour Some Sugar on Me" by Def Leppard
"I Want Your Sex" by George Michael
"Turnin' Me Up" by BJ the Chicago Kid
"Love Sex Magic" by Ciara
"Like a Virgin" by Madonna
"Can't Wait" by Jill Scott
"Fade Into You" by Mazzy Star
"Luv" by Tory Lanez
"Need You Tonight" by INXS
"Lake by the Ocean" by Maxwell
"Do You Mind" by the xx

"I Do" by Musiq Soulchild
"Sexual Healing" by Marvin Gaye
"I'll Make Love to You" by Boyz II Men
"French Kiss" by Lil Louis
"Sexy MF" by Prince
"Closer" by Nine Inch Nails
"The Sweetest Taboo" by Sade
"I Just Wanna Make Love to You" by Etta James
"Lollipop" by Lil Wayne
"Jeepster" by T. Rex
"Make You Feel My Love" by Bob Dylan
"Lovesong" by Adele

#LOVESEXMUSIC

INGREDIENTS

2 smartphones with Spotify

an appreciation for a good song

LIKE SEX, MUSIC IS ONE OF THE UNIVERSAL joys of life. Sometimes they coincide; there's nothing new about using music to get in the mood or as a background enhancer when you're getting it on. But what about music as foreplay? Seriously stimulating, tension-mounting, mind-melting foreplay. This week, Spotify is going to help you get lucky. More specifically, your astute ear and ability to set the right tone by taking control is going to get you lucky. You're going to communicate through songs, using music to do most of the talking for you. Or at least the texting.

If you're both audiophiles, then you've got it made. If you're not, well, who doesn't love music?

All you need is the Spotify app on your phones; before you get started, make sure she has it on hers. Thanks to the Teaser you sent earlier this morning or the day before, she's already been alerted than you have something planned.

You're first text isn't a text. Pick a song to share and send it to her, without any words or hints. It should have sentimental element to it. Set the tone with a song you know she's familiar with. Maybe it's the first song you danced to together or the one that was playing the night you met. Start romantic, then gradually heat things up to the highly charged.

Playing DJ might not be your thing, so I've got you covered! See the playlist at the end of this seduction. Ideally, each song you pick is personal on some level—or it's a tune you *know* inspires her to sway her hips and feel her sultry side. Or get in touch with her inner freak.

Maybe she'll pick up on the game instantly. If she writes back something like, *As, I love that song!*, then spell it out. Text her: *Now it's your turn to send a song back to me. xox*

And by the way, be ready for a sex date on Saturday night.

SEND HER THE TEASER!

TYPE THE LINK BELOW. CASE SENSITIVE.

101nights.com/ LoveSexMusic

FOR HIS EYES ONLY

NO. 32

WAH-WAH-WOW!

101 NIGHTS OF GREAT SEX

on her nightie: *straighten up the bedroom*. Whoa, wait, don't toss this page! I'm not saying you have to change the sheets or actually *clean* the place. Just make the bed. Put your stuff in the closet. Light a few candles.

It won't be long before your girl is happy and aroused and sprawled in bed. Slip down between her thighs and work some magic with your tongue, and then, after a few minutes, reach for your gift bag, hidden under the bed. Hold it high, and smile. You don't even have to say a word. Just reach in and slide out *one* of your new toys. Pop the end into your mouth to get it wet, and then turn it on low. Ahhh. What a lovely sound. Every woman adores it. Don't apply the buzzer straight to the clit; it's much too soon for that. Instead, draw a loop around her whole vulva, slowly circling in toward her lips. Alternate between your tongue and the toy, gradually ramping up the intensity of your action. Take one of her labia into your mouth while stroking the other with the vibe. Tease her. And then…

Hold up your gift bag again. Let her watch you reach in and pull out the *other* toy. She's thinking, "Wow, this is getting *interesting*." Turn it low, like the first vibe, and stroke her with it. Stroke her with the other one again. *Then stroke her with both.* Hold them parallel and glide them alongside her clitoris, just for a moment. She might gasp; the sensation is intense. Turn up the speed on both machines, and use them to draw patterns on her.

Your new friend, *constructive interference*, is about to swagger into the room and help make things crazier. Speed up the vibes, but tune them so they are not quite on the same note. Feel the beat? That wah-wah sound is even more intense when you feel it pounding your hand. The slow pulse of interference is more than noise; it's a visceral shake—and you're about to use that power to shake up your lover.

Press the two toys against her on either side of her swollen clit. Send that powerful *wah-wah* beat through her. Slide the toys up and down her lips. Put one of them inside again, just two inches deep, right where her G-spot is now screaming for relief; put the other one outside, near her clitoris, and *oh… my… god*—the pleasure is strong, overwhelming… bigger than anything she has felt before.

The beat of the fighting vibrations carries her to a place where she can no longer control her body. A place where she can only curl her toes, arch her back, and ride along with the pulses. A place where she might say dirty things and not even remember them. A place she'll want to visit again and again, and take you with her…

NO.32 WAH-WAH-WOW!

INGREDIENTS

2 one-piece vibrators with adjustable speed controls (Corn's recommendation: buy two "Breeze 3-speed Power Bullets" at thepleasurechest.com only $14.95 a piece)

1 gift bag

Head's Up!
One of the vibrators purchased for this seduction can also be used for Heels on a Dash, Tongue and Cheek, Light Her Up, and Clit Bait.

SEND HER THE TEASER!

TYPE THE LINK BELOW. CASE SENSITIVE.

101nights.com/Wah-Wah-Wow

IF YOU'VE EVER TUNED A GUITAR tuned a guitar or ridden in a twin-engine boat, you're familiar with the *wah-wah* effect that happens when two sounds are close in pitch, but not exactly the same. It's the sound of two notes fighting each other, and it's called *constructive interference.*

I'm no acoustic engineer, so I'm not interested in explanations of sine waves and amplitudes; I'd rather talk about orgasms. Or, more precisely, use science to help you create [drum roll]... The World's Most Powerful Orgasm. (*"BWAH-HAH-HAH hah-hah-hah!"* cackled the horny mad scientist. *"Oh, no"* cried the helpless maiden, *"Not another powerful orgasm!"*)

You will need *two* vibrators to create this extraordinary treat. They should be one-piece units—easy to handle, like drumsticks. *Important:* they must have an *adjustable speed controller*, not just an on-off switch. Before your night begins, test your vibes and make sure you can tune them to the same pitch. (As always, wash them thoroughly. That's just good sex-toy manners!) Put them into a gift bag, and if you want to make an impression—and impressions *count*—use a velvet pouch.

Early in the week send your honey the Tease. Then follow it up with a text asking her on a date. Once the time is set, then make your dinner plans. It can be fancy or a simple takeout dinner. The important thing is that you plan *something* rather than nothing. Simple, but it's the difference between romance and being taken for granted. Or, to put it another way, it can be the difference between "Let's go to sleep" and "Let's screw like weasels."

Meanwhile, here's another trick that makes a woman feel like taking off her sweats and putting

NO. 33

THE GOOP EFFECT

vibrator. She also understands the importance of experimenting to keep things interesting—and there's no better place than an adult store to find fresh new ways to experiment with your honey.

This week, you're going to turn a trip to a sex store into a bonding activity. Maybe it'll make you blush. Good! Your sheepish blush will have nothing on the orgasmic flush that comes as your reward after your little excursion. Tell your man you want to go shopping…but not to the mall. No, this is a shopping spree he's going to want to be a part of! Wherever you live, every town has at least one sexy shop and you're going to find it! Most of these stores are open late, so it could be an ideal post-dinner excursion after you've both had a couple of drinks. Hey, a little liquid courage never hurt.

(If the real-life shopping experience doesn't appeal to you, you can always explore online. Spend the day perusing and send your man links to potential purchases, from the semi-innocent to the wickedly wild, and at the end, pick one and surprise him with it.)

Who cares if you're giggling like a couple of kids?! Looking at all this X-rated stuff together—from tickle feathers and silk blindfolds to vibrators in all shapes and sizes to costumes to help unleash new characters—is a hoot. **It's also foreplay…with a function.** As Gwyneth herself has said: "Whether tantra or BDSM or threesomes or vanilla are your thing will never be the point—knowing yourself, and all your options and how to ask for and pursue what feels good to you is."

As you explore, you're going to discover what you're both into, as you get hotter and hotter for each other by the minute. Looking at all this sexy stuff will unleash your libidos, along with your imaginations. Maybe you didn't even realize you love the look of a hot-pink collar around your neck. Or you had no idea your honey has always fantasized about seeing you in a naughty nurse uniform…or a bondage harness.

The final part of the challenge: You can't leave without buying *at least* one item! It doesn't matter what, as long as it's something you agree on—that you'll want to try the *second* you get home. Tie each other up, let him work a new toy on you, channel a dangerously sultry character: Whatever you choose, put it to good use—and make each other come and come again.

You just purchased something priceless: A new and unexpected fantasy that's sure to unleash countless more erotic adventures!

NO. 33 THE GOOP EFFECT

INGREDIENTS

1 adult boutique

1 sexy shopping companion

"This is not just another sex book...Sounds simple but the anticipation and mystery makes even the smallest gestures pretty thrilling."

-GWYNETH PALTROW

I was walking on the Santa Monica boardwalk when I found out Gwyneth Paltrow had just raved about my book. Even better, she was actually *using* it in her own bedroom, to spice up her sex life! Turns out that was just the beginning of what would come to be a great collaboration.

Since launching Goop in 2008, Gwyneth has been a groundbreaking force for women's sexual empowerment in her own right. From sex-positive guides, designed to help you explore uncharted territories, to boundary-pushing toy recommendations to articles like, "*How to Have More Sex*," Goop has championed the importance of expanding your sexual horizons (and try things you wouldn't have ever expected) for over a decade now. So when Gwyneth asked me to contribute to Goop's new book, The Sex Issue, I jumped at the chance. Packed with fresh ideas, wisdom and anecdotes, it's going to help take your sex life to places you hadn't expected. Which is what I'm all about!

Of course, I mean *figurative* places like new heights of ecstasy, transcendent worlds of pleasure, and unprecedented levels of connection with your partner. But I also mean *literal* places...like your local adult boutique!

Gwyneth has always been one to be vocal about recommending her preferred sex toys, which have included organic lube, a stylish Agent Provocateur whip, and even a super-decadent 24-karat gold

SEND HIM THE TEASER!

TYPE THE LINK BELOW. CASE SENSITIVE.

101nights.com/
TheGoopEffect

NO. 34

HEADS OR TAILS

- Kiss her neck while reaching around front to tweak her nipples.

- Slip one hand between her legs while massaging her neck with the other.

- Hover over the front of her thighs while kissing her bottom.

- Press your fingers against her clit, then run your tongue in one slow swipe from the base of her spine all the way up to her neck. If that doesn't turn her knees to jelly, check her pulse!

After a while, move her to the bed, face up, arms bent (and probably shaking) at her sides. Keep counting every time she trembles enough to knock a coin off her wrists, while you:

- Glide your hands up her legs while sucking her toes.

- Gently pinch a nipple while running your tongue from hip to hip.

- Stretch her nipple taut. This makes it stiff and immobile and so, so sensitive; she'll gasp when you lick it.

Here's a technique that may bounce those nickels off your ceiling! Gently press your palm into her *Mons Veneris*, the little bulge where her pubic hair grows, or would grow, if she's bare. Pull her flesh in small, slow circles with your palm. As the skin of her mons slides around, it stretches all those lovely, sexually charged nerves in her lips and clitoris. After half a minute, stop your tender tugging, lift your fingers, and tap them against her vaginal lips. Tap...tap...tap... lightly, once or twice per second.

Ten taps, then rub your palm in ten circles. Tap again, then massage with your hand. Repeat until she melts. I call it *Palm Reading, Laura Corn Style*. Because it's easy to read her reaction to your palm; she'll be gasping and moaning and visibly struggling to keep those nickels in place.

Game over. How many times has she dropped them? "*Oooh, that's the number of favors you're going to do for me,*" you whisper as you climb on top of her, filling her soaked and aching, desperate-for-climax little hole. "One coin, one sexual favor. You're in debt right now, but don't worry. You get to knock the nickels off me next time..." Until then, you've got some decisions to make. You obviously won, so what are you going to claim for your reward? Maybe you should toss a coin:

Heads or tails?

INGREDIENTS

1 dresser or desk

1 pillow

1 text message asking her to bring 2 nickles to the bedroom

anything that will make her quiver

SEND HER THE TEASER!

TYPE THE LINK BELOW. CASE SENSITIVE.

101nights.com/
HeadsOrTails

HOW MANY EROGENOUS ZONES DO YOU HAVE? Other than *that* one, I mean. (Although I have to admit, that's one heckuva great zone.)

Besides the obvious places, the human body can feel pleasure in dozens of spots. With the right attention, almost any inch of skin can be tantalized, tickled and turned on. This week, you're going to devote an evening to finding as many ways as possible to make her quiver.

She's going to show up at the bedroom door wondering why your text asked her to bring **two shiny nickels**. "Oh, it's the price of admission to my new game," you can tell her, with a wink, as you take the coins. "It requires a bit of skin, though..." Help her undress, and once she's down to her panties and bra, put a pillow on the dresser and invite her to bend over it. She should be quite comfortable like this: legs straight and slightly apart, arms and head resting on the pillow. Make sure her forearms are facing up, exposed. "Here's the game. I'm going to put one nickel on the back of each wrist. Let's see how long you can keep them there!" Ah, now that's a challenge! She has to stay perfectly still—while you use every erotic trick you know to make her tremble. Count out loud every time a coin falls and has to be put back in place. *One, two, three, four.* With each rising number, so is her tension level.

Now touch her. Touch her everywhere, and always in at least two places at once. Sometimes you'll use the *Hover Massage*, a technique where your hands grazes only her ultra-fine body hair, sending tingles of static electricity into her skin. Try this:

- Caress her face with your fingertips while your lips graze her ears.

NO. 35

NOT THAT INNOCENT

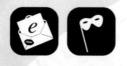

drop the pillow and stick out his hands. Tie a knot around his wrists, and instruct him to raise his hands high. Throw the other end of the rope over the top of the door, and then tie it to the doorknob on the other side. Now unbutton, unsnap, unzip.

You can do whatever you feel like. He wants you to be in charge. Sure, he might jump a bit when you tweak his nipple, or slide an ice cube down his bare buttocks, but there's nothing he can do to stop you. More to the point, he won't even try.

Is he being a good little submissive? Then give him his reward. Kneel on the pillow in front of him. Bring his penis to your mouth and rub it against your lips. Feel him tremble when you glide your tongue all the way around the crown.

"You love when I do this, don't you?" Oh, yes, he certainly does. Pull him into your mouth and suck him like a Popsicle on a hot day.

"You'd like me to keep doing this until you make a mess all over my lips, wouldn't you?" Oh, yeah, YES please don't stop.

"You want me to suck a little harder, don't you?" YES yes yes yes, ohhh, yes please.

"You want to buy me a new Gucci bag and matching wallet, don't you?" Oh, yes, please—huh??

Just kidding about that last part. (Or not.) But keep that same attitude in mind all night.

You make the rules. You are in control. And when you have finally allowed him relief, and release, you still get to tell him exactly what you want, and how to do it. Maybe more than once.

Your final command? Tell him to find a way to hang that lovely long rope permanently in the closet. That way, he will see it every day—and remember who's the boss.

INGREDIENTS

1 pillow

1 8-foot section of smooth nylon rope

high heels

lingerie

a wicked smile

no fear

"Oops, you think I'm in love / That I'm sent from above / I'm not that innocent"

BRITNEY SPEARS, *"OOPS... I DID IT AGAIN"*

I just *love* using props for a seduction. They really set the mood. As every woman knows, a few well-chosen accessories can bring out a character you didn't even know you had inside you. You and your guy might both be surprised by how much you enjoy meeting your inner dominatrix this week.

Give him a long wet kiss, with just a hint of bite, and whisper your instructions. *"Meet me in the bedroom tonight at 8:30 exactly. Be ready for anything. And bring a pillow."*

When he shows up, let him get a good long look at you. You're hot: nightclub makeup, lingerie, the highest heels you can walk on. And then there's that one little extra surprise draped over your shoulders. It's a rope. The silky smooth nylon kind, several feet long.

Do you hear a nervous crack in his voice? Did his eyes get a little wider when he saw you twirling the ends of your rope?

Good. He needs to know that you are in command tonight, starting with your first orders: Tell him to

SEND HIM THE TEASER!

TYPE THE LINK BELOW. CASE SENSITIVE.

101nights.com/
NotThatInnocent

NO. 36

LEATHER KISSES

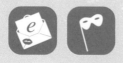

side slightly course, the other butter-smooth. Draw it snug against her face for the overwhelmingly sensual aroma. Bite her nipples through the tender hide.

Instruct her to lay face-down on the bed and, as she stretches out, straddle her back facing her deliciously bare bottom. Massage her thighs and calves. Part her cheeks with your dangerous new toy; trail your fingers between her legs. Is she wet? Is she soaking the tanned skin? Now ask her to turn over; spread her legs wide. Take the very end of your belt and dip it inside her. Get it soaked with her nectar. Place the tip squarely over her clitoris and, with only a light squeeze, gently slide it off. The slick friction, the pressure, the exquisite pop as her clit comes free from it's leather restraint will have it singing. Do it again. And again, faster and firmer. Her moans will let you know how to pop her pussy. Some women like strong pops and others, light strokes, but believe me; for most women, getting their pussy spanked is on a whole other level of hot! Each soft snap of leather on her flesh pushes her closer to the edge. Alternate with light strokes from your fingers and strong licks from your tongue. Make it quicker, and wetter, and when she explodes, press the leather up against her steaming lips. Let her drench them with her honey.

Now, what are you going to do with a belt that carries the very faint aroma of sex? Well, if she pulls it out of the closet for you one evening — it's a sure bet she doesn't want you to get dressed for dinner.

no.36 LEATHER KISSES

INGREDIENTS

1 leather belt (or riding crop)

WHAT IS IT ABOUT LEATHER THAT MAKES IT so fascinating? A woman looks totally hot in a leather miniskirt. A man in black leather strikes us as powerful, even foreboding. Our fantasies are often not of exposed skin, but of a *second* skin made of soft, supple leather.

If she doesn't appreciate the erotic power of leather yet, you're about to open up a whole new world. Start by sending her the Teaser the morning of your seduction. When the evening rolls around, tell her she's in for a treat. Let your flirting turn to touching and when she's all warmed up, lead her into the bedroom.

Then make a dramatic move. Yank off your leather belt, grab it by the ends, and rope her in. Pull her hard against you for a kiss. Slip the strap down her back, stopping every few inches to cinch it in, especially when you've got it tight against her butt.

As you slowly undress her, use your belt like a silk scarf, dragging it across each inch of her flesh, one

SEND HER THE TEASER!

TYPE THE LINK BELOW. CASE SENSITIVE.

101nights.com/
LeatherKisses

NO. 37

CYBORGASM

This Saturday, you're going to wake up a little earlier than normal and set up a scene of your own; you, naked in bed, with your laptop (or smartphone) playing the sultry sounds of porn. Lie back, place your laptop on your tummy or next to you, and hit the video clip you selected earlier. Girl-on-girl can be super-sensual, or opt for something rougher: whatever makes you feel all tingly. You can add a sexy twist by casually texting him earlier in the week, asking his top fantasy category: *Lesbian? Amateur? Big Booty?* He'll probably be thinking, "How about all three?" But mainly, he's going, "It's so hot she just asked me that. What's she got up her sleeve this time?!" He'll find out soon enough, although when he wakes up Saturday, he's going to think he's still dreaming.

First, he'll hear the unfamiliar moans and gasps—intermixed with your own, which he'll suddenly find sexier than ever. Then he'll open his dazed eyes to see you, writhing around, pinching your nipples and caressing yourself under the covers. What a delicious sight! You've just created a dream come true, and he's going to want to jump right in. Roll on over to him, put the laptop on his belly or right next to him, and let him feel how excited you are, as you ride slowly up and down his thigh and kiss and nibble his neck.

You might expect him to be staring at the wild scene on the screen, but I have a feeling he won't be able to take his eyes off you. And just when he thinks it can't get any better, it does. Pull back the covers, position yourself on all fours and raise your ass in the air like your in the throes of heat. You're his own personal porn star and you want him right now.

You know where you're headed; it's only natural to go downtown and give him the full treatment. You're going to move seductively and *sloooowly* backwards, trailing your tongue down his body as you go.

Start by moving your tongue round in circles at the very sensitive head of his penis. Do it quickly—it'll drive him crazy. At the same time, one hand will be sliding up and down his shaft in twisty circles while the other is gently massaging that invisible line between his balls and his anus—it's rich in nerve endings and it's a gold mine when it comes to giving him a supremely intense orgasm.

Welcome to wonderland, created by you. You'll be looking up at him with a naughty glint in your eye as you suck and lick and wave your ass in the air. His eyes will be hovering between the sexy images in front of him and the living sex star in his bed giving him the blowjob of a lifetime.

The grand finale of your personal performance isn't going to be a long time coming. When it does, expect a full-body orgasm that will have him shaking from head to toe. He might be worn out before the day's even really started, but it's so worth it. He'll be beaming all the way to Monday. And if he's never been a morning person, you can bet he'll be an early riser from now on.

NO. 37 CYBORGASM

INGREDIENTS

1 laptop (or smartphone)

1 sexy video clip

1 pair of earbuds (optional)

1 evolved and seXXXy woman

SEND HIM THE TEASER!

TYPE THE LINK BELOW. CASE SENSITIVE.

101nights.com/Cyborgasm

"I LIKE THE PRETTY PORN. IT'S HOT! VINTAGE VIVID IS GOOD PORN!...IT'S JUST SEX."

-Lisa Rinna

Are you ready for an amazing statistic? And I mean *amazinggg*! It might shock you, but who knows? You might be in this very group! One out of *every three women* regularly watch porn. And the number is rising, right along with our orgasms. Surprising, right? Then again, porn has gone from taboo from mainstream, and for good reason. Not only do 31% of women enjoy some racy screen time every now and again, women are more likely to watch it for *longer* (over a minute more than men each time, to be exact).

While going solo is all good, it's a fact that couples who watch porn together *stay* together. Believe it or not, it makes for a steamy bonding session—it's a fantasy escape *and* a stress reliever. Studies show it also helps give women the confidence to ask for what they want in the bedroom. Not that you need any help in that department!

If you've never watched sexy erotica with your man then, trust me, you're going to both be over the moon with this one. I know what some of you are thinking: "No way, Corn!" If you've never watched porn because of your religious beliefs, I feel you. Your values come first, as you well know, so toss this one aside and rip open a brand-new seduction.

But if you haven't because you're shy or "not that kind of girl," then this is a must-try. I'm giving you permission! And for those of you in that growing 31%, good for you.

Only I'm willing to bet you've never watched it like this before. Not only are you and your man going to indulge in some on-screen heat together, get this; he's going to wake up and find *you* watching porn right in front of him. It's going to make for what I like to call a Cyborgasm.

FOR HER EYES ONLY

NO. 38

COWBOY
DREAMS

101 NIGHTS OF GREAT SEX

Giddy up, baby! And hang on tight, because you and your man are in for a very wild ride with this assignment. He's not going to know what hit him when you take the reins, hop on board and give him the ride of his life.

Start out in panties, bra and a pair of boots. Riding boots if you've got 'em. Silky, sensuous gloves are a great idea, too. He'll love the way the leather and the silk feels in combination over his skin.

Now, position yourself over him while he's lying naked on his back. The first move is a slow, easy ride—just climb on top for a bit of Basic Cowgirl. You on top, him down below—and just slide your sexy panties along his member until he's practically bucking beneath you.

Sexily slip off your panties for this next great ride, the Bucking Butterfly. Slide down his long pole and part your lips with your finger to give him the world's best erotic eye candy. If you're wearing gloves, you can stroke him at the same time for a silky treat.

All this riding is sure to make you both hungry, so take a break for a yummy Banana Split. First, it's time to slip out of your bra and show him those amazing breasts of yours. Then slip one leg behind his, burrow his penis inside you and ride him one more time.

He's going to love being your stallion in that position, and you'll love the feel of him rising up to meet you with each thrust.

Final position? Back to the basics of course. This time, ride him for real with Basic Cowgirl. He'll be watching your face and your luscious body as you slide on over him, and put him through his paces. Speed up until the two of you are nearly galloping along—headed right toward ecstasy.

Yee-haw!

INGREDIENTS

illustrations from
Dr. Sadie's book,
Ride 'Em Cowgirl

1 pair of cowboy boots

bra and panties

1 cowboy hat (optional)

1 pair of leather gloves
(optional)

ONE OF MY FAVORITE AUTHORS, SADIE ALLISON, has created this night just for us! She's got some great positions and toys that target the G-spot and these Cowgirl moves do just that.

You, in bra and panties. Boots and gloves are a nice addition if you have them. And a sexy cowboy hat never hurts!

1. Starting position: Basic Cowgirl

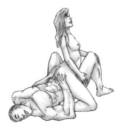

2. Next move: Bucking Butterfly

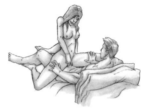

3. Next move Banana Split

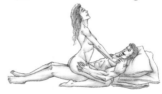

4. Next move Basic Cowgirl

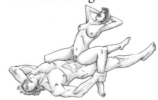

SEND HIM
THE TEASER!

TYPE THE LINK BELOW. CASE SENSITIVE.

101nights.com/
CowboyDreams

NO. 39

SHE'S OUT OF CONTROL

Go start the music, light some candles, arrange some pillows. But every time you finish a task, walk up to her and touch her, caress her, kiss her. Unzip this, unbutton that. Lead her, bound and blindfolded, through the slowest and most sensuous strip tease of her life. This time, though, it's you who is doing the teasing.

Finally, it's time to free her hands and bring her to your special Altar of Eros: a pile of pillows—including the one she brought, of course—laid on the floor at the foot of the bed. Resting at its center: electric magic. Possibly the greatest invention of the century; a vibrator, charged and ready for action.

Instruct her to kneel, facing the bed and straddling the pillows, and adjust the toy so that it is in just the right place. Sit on the edge of the bed directly in front of her. Let her watch, wide-eyed and aroused, as you slowly squeeze and stroke your swelling erection. "And now, you have a very important job to do. It will demand your total concentration and focus. You must take this"—the stiffening erection now rubbing against her face, sliding across her lips—"and make it feel just as good… as that…"

Turn on the vibrator. Set the remote control to slow, at first; it will be more than enough to make her quiver. Now, vary the speed. Slowly notch it up, accelerating the cycle of arousal. Chase that delicious buzz from her lips to your erection to the controller to the toy to her pulsing little clit and straight up her electrified spine, around and around until she explodes, with your own orgasm not far behind.

I have a prediction to make. The next time she's with her friends and they start to complain about the way their men monopolize the remote control, I bet your sweetie will simply smile and say, "Maybe, they just don't know how to use it right…"

NO. 39 SHE'S OUT OF CONTROL

INGREDIENTS

Several candles

Hot music

1 long silk scarf or blindfold

1 remote control vibrator

1 assertive text message (in which you instruct her to bring 1 large pillow and 1 wooden hanger to the bedroom at a designated time)

Two short lengths of nylon rope

HEAD'S UP!
The remote control vibrator purchased for this seduction can also be used for Popping Her Clutch, Light Her Up, Position of Submission, and WAH-WAH Wow.

EQUAL SCHMEQUAL. Tonight, you will be Master; she will be your servant. And she will learn the intensely erotic pleasures of sexual submission.

Your roles must be established as soon as she meets you at the bedroom door. As Commander, you are charming and pleasant, but give no more information than she needs. Why did she bring the large pillow, as spelled out in your text? Why the sturdy wooden coat hanger? "Oh, you'll see," you say slyly and smoothly. "Or, actually, you won't see. I don't want to spoil the surprise."

At this point, you pass a long silk scarf across her eyes and tie it behind her head. Ask her to hold the hanger, gripping the ends, then—while telling her how lovely she is, and how much you've been thinking of her—tie her wrists to the hanger.

Gently press her back to the bedroom door. Lift her arms over her head, and then hook the hanger over the top of the door. Caress her; kiss her neck. "Wha…what are you doing?" she'll undoubtly ask. "Why…whatever I want to. And, oh, there doesn't seem to be anything you can do about it, does there?" Squeeze her nipple, kiss her face. Tell her to be a good girl, to do exactly as her Master says, and she'll get a great big surprise. "I have a few things to do… and I want you to stay right here, where I can… mmm, well… play with you."

SEND HER THE TEASER!

TYPE THE LINK BELOW. CASE SENSITIVE.

101nights.com/
ShesOutofControl

NO. 40

FANTASY SUITE

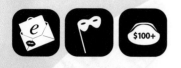

you on vacation, at parties, candidly laughing and maybe even in bed: They should be all around you. You probably have a lot of great photos of the two of you in your phone. Get a few new ones printed, then nicely matted and framed.

Now for the other important items every bedroom needs to be a place where you want to be...and want to be taken.

The first is obvious: It's a set of nice sheets with a soft, inviting duvet on top busy pattern will detract from what's really supposed to be going on in bed.

Next, nothing sets the mood more than candles – and nothing makes you feel sexier than the right lighting. I've been collecting electric candles for years, and I love them. They're clean and turn on in a flash. Plus, you want to light up your sex life. Not burn down the house!

Music is just as important. A single wireless speaker on your nightstand is a game-changer. Which sounds do you find most seductive? Whether it's smooth R&B or thrashing rock 'n' roll, sexy music is so subjective.

Now you need a special place for all your playtime tricks and treats. That's right, a toy box, but one for grownups. Pick out one that possibly has a lock on it (a simple shoebox works, too), keep it somewhere easy to access, and fill it with all your favorite naughty playthings, from vibrators and dildos to handcuffs and whips to wigs and costumes – whatever strikes your fantasy-inspiring fancy.

Once you've completed your makeover, it's time for the grand unveiling. The bed is inviting, candles are flickering, music is playing low, and photos of the two of you adorn the walls. You've got the place to yourselves and time to enjoy the space and each other.

Place your naughty toy box in the middle of the bed. Lead your man into the room, and let him look around in awe. Explore the box together. Then explore each other. Play dress up, if you're in the mood. Let him use your vibrator on you, or handcuff you to the bedpost. Pull out some of the tricks you've learned from other seductions! Christen the sheets with your naked bodies. Kiss him deeply, while he holds you in his arms. Wrap your legs around him and feel the heat of your bodies against each other. Ultimately, this bedroom makeover is about the two of you in the orgasmic microcosm you've created.

Your bedroom isn't just a place to sleep anymore. It's your own private seduction hideaway, hidden right in plain sight.

Home, sweet home!

INGREDIENTS

1 new set of bedding

4-8 electric candles
(start collecting now–you
can never have enough!)

1 Bluetooth speaker

1 box, preferably with
a lock

MAYBE IT'S MIRANDA HOBBES OF *Sex and the City* who says it best: "I'm trying to change my bed karma. I figure if I make my bed a place I really want to be, others will feel the same," she announces, as she makes her bed with fresh new sheets, continuing. "If you build it, he will come." Miranda's on to something here. Except she's forgetting one important detail: You'll come, too!

It's time for a bedroom makeover, but this isn't your typical design revamp. You're going to convert your boudoir from a functional place into a sensual sanctuary. I can't tell you how many couples tell me their bedroom isn't a place they want to have sex. Between gym equipment, pet toys, kids' things and the physical chaos that comes with leading a busy life, the beauty of the bedroom is *buried*. This seduction lies the foundation for countless other seductions in this book. It might be a little expensive, but it's worth every penny. Not only will it improve the quality of your life; it improves the quality of your sex life.

Start by looking around your room, and be objective. Do the colors make you feel more stressed than serene? Is there needless clutter lying around? Pair down and put away! This isn't just about eliminating the junk and keeping what sparks joy (thank you, Marie Kondo). It's about investing in what sparks *orgasms*! If you have photos of your kids sprinkled around, get... them...out. You might not believe this, but they're preventing you from having sex. *I'm not kidding.*

Just like erotic art serves as what I like to call a *subliminal seducer,* pictures of other family members and even friends translates to "no-sex zone." The only people who should be smiling back at you are of you and your sweetie. Pictures of

SEND HIM THE TEASER!

TYPE THE LINK BELOW. CASE SENSITIVE.

101nights.com/
FantasySuite

NO. 41

DIRTY 5

Text 3

"Make sure you're wearing those panties I like. Don't worry about a bra."
She's not just curious by now. The anticipation is killing her.

Text 4

"Tonight is the night! Be prepared for my text after 8pm. The Dirty Five is happening."
Those favorite panties of hers just got damp. She's raring to go and so are you.

Text 5

"Meet me in the guest bathroom in 10 minutes. Bend over the sink with your panties on."

OMG! In her head, she's 25 again and she's heading out to that place in the parking lot behind the restaurant where you used to go in your courting days.

When you finally walk into the bathroom—boom! You're going to see her splayed over the sink, offering her butt up to you. Just stand and admire that incredible view for a few moments while you stroke that growing erection of yours. Then, be concise and to the point. Tell her the Dirty Five means only five minutes of sex. Tell her, "You've got me for five minutes—I'm going to set my phone. So make the most of this."

You're going to hear her moan when she hears that *masterful* tone. Set your phone with the alarm and put it in a place where you can still see it—if you want to check in on how much time you have left. Then with a "Ready, set, go!" slap her legs apart. Run your hands over her those sexy panties, feel how wet she is. She'll want you to take them off and finally you will. Run your hands through her hair, pull it playfully, especially if you know she likes that.

Then turn her into that dirty girl you know she wants to be. Tell her to spit in your hand and then take that spit and rub it on her pussy. It's a good idea to have some lube handy. Women take longer to build up to arousal than men, plus, if she's used to a lot of foreplay, she might feel it's a pressure to get wet so quickly. Make her pussy really oily and juicy and tease her clit with your hands. You can afford to spend at least two of those five minutes playing with her pussy. You want to get her really turned on. She already is totally excited—especially because she knows those minutes are ticking away.

Now that she's really slippery, she's going to be desperate to feel your hard cock enter her. But remember to tease her a little—give it to her slowly; one inch at a time and enjoy watching her breasts jiggle and her face moan with ecstasy in the mirror you probably have over the sink. Thanks to the mirror, you'll also be able to watch yourself getting busy on her from behind—and damn, you look good. By this time, you're both hot and sweaty and you don't have much time left—the urgency of it all is so EXCITING! You can see the countdown on the face of your phone. Let her know time is almost up: "You ready for me, baby?"

You're going to shoot and she's going to shudder and you're both going to feel so wide-awake afterwards. That post-fuck afterglow smile is going to be pasted all over your faces for the next couple of days. And the best thing is that you now have a secret code for when you want five minutes of hot sex. All you say is, "You up for a 'Dirty Five?'" And yes, she is!!!

NO. 41 DIRTY 5

INGREDIENTS

5 teasy texts

1 bottle of lube or regular kitchen oil

1 masterful man

"I want you and I want you right now!"

Remember how often you used to say a variation on that line in the sizzling-hot early days of your relationship? And then the years went by and kids came along? Suddenly, it wasn't so easy to have that intense quickie up against the kitchen wall or in the car on Monday morning when you were supposed to be driving to work.

Well, I'm pleased to say that the good old "I gotta have you now!" quickie is going to reappear in your life this week. Forget soft lighting and flickering candles for now. They're all well and good, but *creative* quickies actually play a crucial role in your sex life. They're exciting, super-energizing, and they have the power to re-light that spark in your relationship by proving you still get hard and wet for each other after all these years. And they're especially important for HER because when a woman feels desired urgently by her lover, it makes her feel sexy and passionate and that's only a good thing, right?

So yes, I'm going to take you back to those spontaneous hot and horny early days. The only difference is this time around you're going to plan the spontaneity or it's not going to happen. You ready to get busy?! Here's what you're going to do:

You're going to send her a series of texts building up to what I'm calling the "Dirty Five," meaning five fast and furious minutes of fast-track pleasure. And five teasing texts.

Here's what your texts might look like:

Text 1
"The Dirty Five is on the menu this week. You feeling hungry?"

That's going to set her juices flowing. She knows you're not talking mac 'n' cheese.

Text 2
"You might want to shave your legs every day this week. You never know when or where it will happen."
She's thinking, "What on earth?"

SEND HER THE TEASER!

TYPE THE LINK BELOW. CASE SENSITIVE.

101nights.com/Dirty5

NO. 42

FORT DO-ME

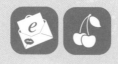

platter to her, she'll see her name on the outside of the card. When she opens it, she'll read something like this:

"Go to the bedroom at 9 PM and put on your PJs. Wait for my call. And then come find me."

Wow! She'll be intrigued and excited, and the night hasn't even started yet. When she goes to the bedroom, you have to head to the living room and break the world record for fastest couch-cushion fort building. (It's a good idea to scout out all your building materials in advance and know where everything is.) Try to finish in under ten minutes, then pick up your cell phone, call your girl, and tell her to come get you.

Ah-ha! The room lights are out! She's wandering down the hall in the near-dark, guided only by a single flickering light coming from the living room. It takes a few seconds to make sense of the scene before her, with cushions and pillows and chairs moved about. The white sheet covering everything up is lit from inside. Judging by the shadows, *you* are also under the sheet, holding a flashlight. You're inviting her inside. It's cozy. There's a blanket on the floor, and pillows to sit on.

If only real camping could be this comfortable. She's enjoying the treats you provided—*ooh! Hot chocolate with marshmallows, yum!*—and she's totally impressed by the effort you put into the whole evening. She's ready to kiss you. She's ready to re-enact some very old summer camp memories. ("There was this one time, in band camp…") But this time, she's ready to take it a little farther; to go from making out to making love. She's ready to get naked and squirmy and wet between the thighs. She's ready to lock her legs around your back and take you deep inside her, ready to push back against your thrusting hips, ready to make you pop.

All because you put in a little extra effort and built her a love nest. All because you made her feel special.

NO. 42 FORT DO-ME

INGREDIENTS

1 platter

1 piece of paper or card stock

1 sofa

2 tall chairs

1 sheet, above

1 blanket, below

1 flashlight

several cushions and pillows

delicious treats

EVERY GUY I KNOW SEEMS TO LIGHT UP when someone stirs the memory of *couch-cushion forts*.

Do you remember how to build one? Sofa cushions turned on their sides to form the walls. Kitchen chairs used as tent poles. A sheet or blanket draped from the chairs to the couch to create a private indoor fortress. For kids, a couch-cushion fort is a perfect little space in which to play. And for consenting adults, it's a perfect little space in which to, ahem, play Doctor.

If there's any lesson I hope you take from this book, it's that *presentation is everything* to a woman. When she sees you go to a little extra trouble to make something special, she gets the message that *she* is special. And that is why this sex date starts with a written invitation on a silver platter.

Okay, maybe not silver. Not everyone gets real silver platters as wedding presents any more. But you're going for true old-school elegance here, the kind of thing they did in the Victorian days, and that requires your finest serving platter. Dig up the one your sweetie uses for Thanksgiving. In the center, place a small white card, folded over and standing up like a tent. When you present the

SEND HER THE TEASER!

TYPE THE LINK BELOW. CASE SENSITIVE.
101nights.com/FortDoMe

NO. 43

LIPSMACKER

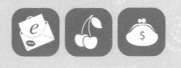

light pecks down her collarbone and around her neck, finishing up with a nibble on the other ear. Don't move towards sex, though. Let her enjoy the anticipation of slow foreplay.

Sometime during the week, go for the We Interrupt This Call Kiss. When she's on her cell with a friend, grab it away and say, *"Could you hold for just a moment?"* Plant a big, passionate kiss on your girl, tell the caller, *"Thank you!"* and hand the phone back. Yes, they will be talking about you for a while. All good.

Friday, add an Ice Cream Kiss to the mix. Put a spoonful of ice cream or other frozen treat in your mouth, then surprise her with your frosty lips. After dinner, be sure to give her a Hershey's Kiss. The actual chocolate candy, I mean. Delicious, and remarkably effective in foreplay.

Come Saturday, launch a fusillade of kisses her way. (If given the opportunity, throw in a Bum Bite! Bite her bare ass before she gets dressed. It will leave her thinking about you every time she sits.) In between one of these mini-makeout sessions, in the morning or early afternoon, pause and tell her to meet you in the living room at sunset for some more kissing surprises.

A gorgeous sight awaits her. When she meets you, the setting sun fills the room with a fiery glow; the light sparkles through a bottle of champagne (of course—*bien sûr!*), and the two flutes next to it. Freshly rinsed strawberries glisten like fat rubies. You've tossed a blanket on the floor, and piled pillows against the sofa to make a comfortable backrest. It's such an easy scene to set, but it's the very essence of romance, the climactic scene of all the best chick-flicks rolled into one. Tell her to go get comfortable and then join you for some Strawberry Kisses.

When she's back, snuggle and make a big presentation of popping the cork. Bubbles dance in the afternoon sunlight as you raise your glass and make a toast to her beauty. Hold a strawberry to her lips; let her take a bite and then… *try to steal it back and replace it with a kiss.* Sip, nibble, and kiss again. Repeat those three steps until clothes begin to disappear.

The French were onto something when they created champagne, which only comes from the region of northeastern France by the same name. And believe it or not, prosecco doesn't offer quite the same effect; champagne is made with a method that yields the best bubbles. The fizz makes magic, and the subtle *brut* dryness is a perfect balance for sweet strawberries (Not to mention the pleasures of champagne oral sex!). The combination inevitably leads to French Kissing. Wet, flirty, deep kisses that let you share the flavor and excitement. But they don't have to be limited to the mouth. Apply a dab of fruit to her nipple; kiss it. Pour a splash of champagne in her bellybutton, and lap it up. Keep moving in that direction. Soon you'll be enjoying what the French call Australian Kissing.

That's a French kiss…*down under.*

NO. 43 LIPSMACKER

INGREDIENTS

1 bottle of champagne

2 pints of strawberries

1 blanket

pillows

SEND HER THE TEASER!

TYPE THE LINK BELOW. CASE SENSITIVE.

101nights.com/
Lipsmacker

WHAT DO WOMEN REALLY WANT?

Men have been asking that question for ages. It used to be obvious—*a little fire, some shelter, and would you be a dear and slay the sabre-tooth tiger stalking the tribe? Thanks so much, honey.*

But ever since settling down and you know, establishing civilization and plumbing, men have become mystified by women. I can tell you what women want, though, because I've talked to over two thousand. It's easy... *more kissing.* In survey after survey, kissing is often considered the biggest turn-on for women. Did you know that when a man kisses a woman, he is actually passing his testosterone onto her? It's this "boost" that puts us in the mood and gets us even more turned on. But alas, women all over the world believe they don't get enough kissing. With one notable exception:

France—the Oral Nation.

The French get *all* the kissing they want. They take pride in making high art out of anything that uses *la bouche*, the mouth. Dinners last hours. *Talking* about dinner lasts hours. And if you ever get a *sommelier* on a rant about French wine—the sipping, tasting, smelling—you're not going anywhere. With all that focus on oral pleasure, it's no surprise that kissing is high on the agenda for the *amoureux* of La République Française.

This week, kissing—in all its wonderful forms—is going to be the focus of your seduction.

Start with Surprise Kisses—delivered out of the blue, randomly, accompanied by a smile and a squeeze. You score lots of points with Surprise Kisses and they require virtually no preparation (other than brushed teeth, plus mints or mouthwash. But you knew that already, didn't you? Of course you did. I'm just saying).

Thursday, give her a Necklace Kiss. Start on the neck, just below her ear, and then plant a circle of

NO. 44

PINK BREAKFAST

to her; she'll love being held as she drifts in and out of that drowsy half-awake state. When she slips back into dreamland, crawl out of bed and head for the kitchen, where you'll make some coffee or tea or some other hot drink. Bring her a cup, but before you present it to her, take a big sip—

And climb under the covers. Way under. Try very hard not to wake her before you run your tongue right across her belly and down to her sweetness.

Wow! What a way to wake up. The drink has heated your mouth and moistened your lips. Your tongue is creating steam everywhere it touches. The hot fluid engorges her, making every lick feel like an orgasm.

She might still be dreaming...sweet dreams, no doubt. But soon she'll come to realize the magic you're making is no fantasy. Don't expect conversation from your little sleepyhead this morning—but a deep sigh and a few moans will let you know you're on the right track.

As for you, enjoy, but I should warn you: a mouthful of hot liquid will also speed up her orgasm and make it twice as intense.

And twice as addictive.

NO. 44 PINK BREAKFAST

INGREDIENTS

1 sleepyhead

A little sleepy head!

WHAT'S THE TASTE OF PASSION?

On radio and in interviews, I've talked to a lot of men over the years. They can all name favorite aromas that put them in the mood for love— flowers, a special perfume, even a certain favorite meal on the stove can trigger hot memories. All men seem to love the smell of a woman's freshly washed hair.

But when it comes to taste, there's just one that's always guaranteed to, um, raise the flag, if you know what I mean. It's the glorious, fragrant, slightly sweet and always highly evocative flavor of your lady's you-know-what. This week, believe it or not, you're going to sneak a bite when your lover isn't looking!

Pick a day when you both can sleep in for a while without interruption. First thing in the morning, encourage her to stay in the sack. Cuddle up close

SEND HER
THE TEASER!

TYPE THE LINK BELOW. CASE SENSITIVE.

101nights.com/
PinkBreakfast

NO. 45

LIGHTS! CAM! ACTION!

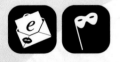

or two. Or stay true to you. It doesn't matter: the heat here is delivered via the barrier of the screens. If he sees you go off to the bedroom, even better. Give him a sly wink and shut the door.

A little before your session, set the mood in the room. Pile pillows behind you, so you can fully recline and prop your computer up in front of you on the bed. Make sure the lighting is just right; placing a lamp with a blue or pink lightbulb behind the monitor will add to the experience. Play some sexy music low in the background. Keep some extra lingerie and maybe a sex toy or two, like a vibrator, off to the side. You might want to make a costume change or even racier mischief part of your show.

Once you're both online, greet him seductively and let him know you're about to play a game. *"Hey, there. What's your name?"* you ask as you suck on your lollipop. This suggestive prop will not only help you ease into the performance, it'll signal to him that it's on, baby—and that you'd much rather have your lips wrapped around something else. *"I'm just so horny right now. I can't help it!"* Play it up and he'll get the idea instantly. Keep going, as you writhe around the bed. Feeling a little shy? Use it! Bite your lip in between licks on your lollipop. A girlish giggle can be particularly enticing. Or get commanding. Tell him how hot it is when he gets hard for you, how much it turns you on to see *him* get turned on.

This isn't just deliciously lascivious entertainment for you both. This is hands-off foreplay at its finest. Well, his hands will be all over you soon enough. But while you're working the cam, I highly recommend getting handsy with yourself. Slip your bra or top off and start to caress your breasts. Give them a squeeze. Turn around while you gaze back at him on the screen and give your booty a nice slap. Work your way down and tug on your panties just to tease him. By now he'll be begging you to pull them to side and play with yourself.

Will you do it? The beauty of the on-screen seduction is that even if you're playing submissive, you're the one in control. He's off somewhere else dying to reach out and touch you, but all he can do is succumb to stroking himself.

To take it up a notch, bring out your toy. You can be the naughty girl you really are when you're all alone, since he's not physically in the room. He's watching you watch yourself. What's so hot about this is that he gets to feel like a voyeur; viewing you with the separation of the computer means he's seeing you with new eyes. And the fact that he can't have you just yet, well, that's what brings it over the edge.

Just make sure he doesn't go *over* the edge before you tell him it's time to take it offline and beckon him to come on in for real sex. Let him know he can have you in real life— that's how badly you're aching for him. Then greet him with plenty of passion; at this point, you're nearly naked or fully nude and raring to go.

Who needs a virtual simulation when you're about to enjoy some real-life stimulation?!

NO. 45 LIGHTS! CAM! ACTION!

INGREDIENTS

2 computers (preferably laptop) with Wifi connections

1 sexy outfit (bonus points for extra outfits or accessories)

1 lollipop

your favorite sex toy or two (optional)

1 babysitter (as needed)

TIP: If you don't have access to two computers, you can perform your "show" with the same results on Facetime with your phones.

SEND HIM THE TEASER!

TYPE THE LINK BELOW. CASE SENSITIVE.

101nights.com/ LightsCamAction

FROM EMAILS TO INSTAGRAM TO FACEBOOK, we spend way too much of our lives staring at screens. So why shouldn't we take full advantage of the technology at our fingertips? We know our computers come with built-in cameras, discreetly positioned on the monitor right above the screen. But did you know those little cameras can function as portals of unspeakable lust and pleasure?

Single people and couples in long-distance relationships spend plenty of time on webcams, but they shouldn't get to have all the online fun. That's right, this week you're going to use your computer to channel your inner webcam superstar and create a private show just for your man. If that sounds intimidating, trust me, once you catch a glimpse of yourself on the screen, not only will you be transported to a virtual fantasyland, you'll feel sexy, liberated, even empowered. I promise! Here's how:

Pick an evening or weekend afternoon when you have the place to yourself. Well *almost* to yourself – more on that in a sec. If you have kids, make sure they are out of the house because this seduction requires the takeover of not one but two rooms! I recommend claiming the bedroom as your domain, since you'll want space to relax. Then take your pick between Skype and Google Hangout; whichever you feel more comfortable using.

Ahead of the big day, after you've made sure your webcam works (just click on the camera icon and if you can see yourself on the screen, you're good to go), shoot your honey a text: *Meet me Saturday afternoon online. Don't be late. I'll be waiting for you. And make sure you're all alone.* Be explicit: Tell him exactly what time to go to a spare bathroom or the living room (somewhere he's got privacy) and where to dial in. *Whoa!* He just got very excited. *Whaaaat? Meet her online?!*

Sign your text off with your made-up cam-girl name, something cheeky and different. Imagine a whole new persona for yourself. You have the power to decide who you want to be, if only for the next hour

NO. 46

KING THONG

She's probably even shaved in, you know, the panty region. Dinner leads to kissing, and groping, and unzipping. Help her get her clothes off—*except for her underwear.* Because now it's time to demonstrate Panty Skill Number Two: the use of panties as a sexual tool. Yes, I mean you can make her come by using her panties, just like you use your fingers or tongue.

Tug on them so they slide across her clitoris and lips. Stroke her through the fabric. I'm telling you, this is hot. You're stirring up erotic high school memories of the days before she dared to go All The Way—steamy make-out sessions, sweaty nights in cars, bumping and rubbing and *almost* doing it. Getting close, and getting really wet.

Keep it up for a while. Press your fingertips against her, finger her, just a little inside, with nothing but a sheer layer of fabric between her and your hand. Now introduce her to a truly wild sensation: Oral sex through her panties. Let her feel the heat of your breath. Nibble. Lick. Take your time. Slide the shiny wet fabric around with your teeth and tongue. Then switch. Come back up for air and pull yourself towards her mouth. Kiss her madly, while fingering her over the now-soaked fabric. Bring her right to the edge of orgasm and keep her there until she's pushing back at you, grinding her underwear against your mouth. Then, when she's just about ready to come—slip the fabric to the side for direct contact. It won't be long before she arches her back and bursts into a toe-clenching orgasm.

And it won't be long before you see *those* panties again, I promise.

INGREDIENTS

1 pair of panties

DON'T THINK OF PANTIES as something that gets in the way of sex. *Think of them as an opportunity to show off your skills.*

Panty Skill Number One: *attention to detail.* Want to know why women spend so much on fancy underwear? Because we expect you to notice. No, it's even more than that. We get turned on when you notice tiny details about us. It makes us feel loved. Desired, and desirable. Horny, even. So this week, find the sexiest panties she owns, the ones she wears on special occasions, and study them. Then impress the crap out of her:

"Hey, baby, you know those panties you have, the really hot black ones with the lace around the legs and the red bow right at the top?" Of course she knows. She's surprised to learn that you know, though. "Well, I want you to wear them tomorrow night." Big leering grin, here. "I have plans for them."

A little later on, send her the Tease. By now she's really intrigued, and looking forward to your date.

SEND HER
THE TEASER!

TYPE THE LINK BELOW. CASE SENSITIVE.
101nights.com/KingThong

NO. 47

P IS FOR PORNSTAR

Knees up, legs apart. Arch your back like you're onstage at a strip club. Sure, you may be nervous, but trust me, your man is *loving* this. Let him see your fingers slide under the edge of your panties. Pull them aside and let him get a full, long view as your stroke your lips and circle your clit. Once you're wet—really wet—slip a finger inside and then—classic porn move here—put your finger in your mouth and suck it.

Glance over between his legs. *"Make that hard for me. I want to see you play with it."* Now go into full Jenna mode. Stroke faster. Pinch your nipples. Breathe hard. If you can, give yourself a big, glorious, shuddering climax. (And if you have to fake it, well, you're in good company...I did, too! But Jenna says she gets off for real. Lucky girl.)

Did he come? A lot of men would, watching their own private sex show. If he hasn't, all the better. You can finish him off. Not with any fancy tricks or coy little licks, oh no—he's way past that point now. What he needs is more of what he's been doing, and every guy has his own particular way of doing it. Did you notice the stroke and the style he was using while he was enjoying your performance? *That's* what you need to do now. Kneel in front of him and give him that same twist, that same pull, that same amount of friction. And when you take him in your mouth, be sure to give him that famous Jenna Jameson doe-eyed gaze; the look that says you're enjoying his orgasm just as much as he is.

Now *that's* how to make love like a pornstar.

NO.47 P IS FOR PORNSTAR

If you opened this seduction before completing #49, Queen V, I highly recommend doing that one first. Otherwise, enjoy!

INGREDIENTS

1 chair

music

a lot of confidence

alcoholic beverage, as needed

IMPORTANT NOTE:
If you opened this seduction before completing #49, Queen V, I highly recommend doing that one first. Otherwise, enjoy!

THIS WEEK'S SEXY SURPRISE COMES TO US courtesy of Jenna Jameson, famed pornstar of the '90s and early 2000s. In 2004, at the height of her career, she published a huge bestseller; *How To Make Love Like A Porn Star* and let me tell you, it's a classic.

One particular chapter really stuck in my head. She painted a scene so erotic that I couldn't shake it, and I knew I would have to recreate it for my own guy. It wasn't just the sex that made it so arousing. It was more about sexual confidence and a big dose of raw boldness. That's the kind of thing I don't always feel in real life. But I always feel great when I can pull it off—even if I have to fake it a little along the way.

You're going to need some courage for this one. (And maybe a drink or two!) Tonight you're a pornstar. Start with a text to get his attention: *Show starts at 8. Meet me in the bedroom.* When the time comes, greet him with a kiss, but don't say a word. Just lead him to a chair you've set up in the bedroom. Music and soft light are a must. Strip to your undies, lie down on the floor directly in front of your man, and then...start to play with yourself.

SEND HIM THE TEASER!

TYPE THE LINK BELOW. CASE SENSITIVE.

101nights.com/
PForPornstar

FOR **HIS EYES** ONLY

NO. **48**

TONGUE & CHEEK

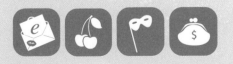

101 NIGHTS OF GREAT SEX

maybe some fruit and toaster waffles. Whatever. Utensils are next to the plate, wrapped in big cloth napkins, just like at a nice restaurant. Now the next part is optional, but for maximum impact, you are wearing an apron. And once you bring the tray to her, it will become clear that under your apron you are wearing...no pants. (If you have kids at home, be a little strategic and change in the bathroom.)

Ha! Yes, your bare butt is hanging out. Because there's nothing like a good belly laugh to start the morning, and I suspect your sweetie will shake the walls with her laughter. But don't stress over the apron if you don't have one; it actually doesn't really matter what you're wearing. It's what you're doing that counts. Her next surprise comes when she unrolls the napkins. One napkin contains a fork and a knife. The other contains, holy cow, is that a...a *vibrator?* Why yes, it is. Fully charged, of course. For dessert.

Kiss her, and feed her, and model your bare-ass apron for her. And now, for the rest of your sunrise surprises. Do all of the following slowly, and multiple times: Put a slice of fruit on her bellybutton and nibble it up. Take a mouthful of ice water or OJ and run your chilled tongue over her nipples. Sip some hot coffee to make your mouth exceptionally warm and wet, and then climb between her parted legs and go down on her. *Oh-hh-hh wow.* That is an incredible feeling. That hot-mouth trick is called "The Velvet Tongue," and it is, in my own personal opinion, the greatest sex move ever invented. Your mileage may vary. But I'll bet your sweetie melts when you bring the heat.

It's been one hell of a memorable morning for her. Sleeping late. Breakfast in bed. A little sugar buzz, a little coffee buzz. And now the ultimate buzz—the vibe, sitting on your serving tray. Use it to alternate with your tongue. Thirty seconds of licking, thirty seconds of buzzing, repeat and repeat. And repeat. Turn up the heat. Kick it up a notch. Show her that you are the Bobby Flay of the bedroom. You've brought new meaning to the name Naked Chef. You are Wolfgang Puck—with a capital F.

Actually, judging by that tent pole propping up your apron, I'd have to say you are really the new Top Chef.

NO. 48 TONGUE & CHEEK

INGREDIENTS

1 table tray

2 cloth napkins

1 apron

1 vibrator

1 weekend morning

breakfast (include something chocolate or sweet)

Head's Up!
The Tongue & Cheek "vibrator" can also be used for Position of Submission, Clit Bait, Light Her Up, and Heels on a Dash.

For a woman, there's a world of difference between good sex and *awesome, tell your girlfriends, look-back-on-it-with-a-smile* sex. And the difference is something that is easy, rewarding and completely in your control. It is this:

A little extra effort.

That's it! You don't have to do it all the time. You don't have to spend a bundle. You simply have to show her, from time to time, that you think she's worth some extra effort. Take it from your old pal Corn, who knows a thing or two about what makes couples happy. You will save yourself a world of aggravation over the years if you just, occasionally, on days that are not Mother's Day or her birthday, prepare Breakfast In Bed. And also why not show your bare ass while you do it.

This weekend, you're going to put just a little more effort into your extra effort. Start by giving away part of your surprise. Tell your sweetie that she can stay in bed on Sunday morning, because you are going to make breakfast and take care of everything. Kids, animals, housework; she won't have to worry about a thing. The morning of, make good on your promise. You don't have to make a feast. (Or a mess!) But remember, with women, presentation counts for a lot. Whether she's told you so or not, she wants to be served. By you.

So when you step into the bedroom, this is what she will see: you carrying a tray with coffee, juice,

SEND HER THE TEASER!

TYPE THE LINK BELOW. CASE SENSITIVE.

101nights.com/
TongueAndCheek

FOR HER EYES ONLY

NO. 49

QUEEN V

Here's what your week's going to look like:

DAY ONE (5 MINUTES):
Take your time. Make sure you're comfortable on the bed or floor, and take the mirror in your hand. If you don't have natural light coming in, you might want to set up a lamp nearby. Get completely naked or at least remove your panties, open your legs, and then just look at that exquisite pussy. Gaze at the color, the shape, touch all the folds. Smell your hands – that's the smell that your guy loves more than anything in the world. Almond oil is useful to have handy. Your fingers will glide over the surface.

DAY TWO (NO TIME LIMIT):
Have a look here at Betty Dodson's actual web site. https://dodsonandross.com/articles/category/vulva-styles You'll see some diagrams and drawings of pussies. Chances are, they differ from yours – and that's one important fact you're going to learn in this vulva exercise. Pussies are all different, but they're all absolutely perfect. Carry on gliding with those oily fingers.

DAY THREE (5 MINUTES):
What's with the "vulva" word, anyway? Well, it turns out that this beautiful word is the correct one for "pussy" because unlike "vagina," it encompasses the whole works: the inner and outer labia, the vagina, the clitoral hood and THE CLITORIS which, don't forget, is our main source of pleasure. So check out each and every part. What does your clitoris look like? Do you need to lift the hood up to see it? What shape do your inner labia make? Can you see an angel? A rose?

DAY FOUR:
I know you're feeling big pussy love by now, so give her a NAME! It can be whatever you feel. In *Sex Drive*, Stephanie names her pussy, Pinky Tuscadero, referring to the Fonz's hell-raising biker girlfriend from *Happy Days* (I call mine the Queen! Because the real Queen Bee–no offense, Beyoncé–is between my legs.) Celebrate the fabulous re-birth by giving your clit some extra attention. You know you love to stroke her and if you're feeling it, *go all the way*! I bet you've never seen yourself come before—I know I never had before I tried this! It's an unforgettable moment, believe me. Plus, it will get you in the mood for Day Five…

DAY FIVE:
Check out an amazing website called OMGYes.com. You're going to watch an incredible group of women doing what you've just done for the past four days—but with the aid of some enticing visuals. Plus, it's a real feel-good thing to see just how at home they are talking about (and showing) their pussies. I highly recommend you subscribing to the site. When your partner chooses the OMGyes! seduction in this book, you're going to watch the Series 2 visuals with him and it's going to be ***the best thing that ever happened to your relationship***.

DAY SIX:
Well-done! You're now a possessor of true pussy power! So take that empowerment and let him in on the act, too. Prop up some pillows, lower the lights, and open your legs. Then send him a text asking him to join you. Get him to sit on the bed and just look at your brand-new pussy that just received a lot of well-deserved love. Trust me: He's going to notice the difference. From here on out, just do what feels right. Listen to your newly tuned-up body. If you're like me, that's probably going to involve a night of making love with wild abandon.

INGREDIENTS

1 small mirror

1 angle poise lamp (optional)

1 bottle of lube or kitchen oil (almond is great)

1 room of your own

1 computer to watch www.omgyes.com

IMPORTANT NOTE:
For all my 101Nights fans, use the code "omgyes.com/101nights" to get a discount.

SEND HIM THE TEASER!

TYPE THE LINK BELOW. CASE SENSITIVE.

101nights.com/QueenV

" When a woman doesn't connect with her pussy, the lights go off inside her—and inside of her family and her world. A woman can't do her job of being a woman without her sensual brilliance engaged. She is working with a 25-watt bulb instead of the 100 watts that are her birthright."

-PUSSY: A RECLAMATION BY MAMA GENA

You know what the most sought-after thing in the world is? Men treasure it. They fight for it. They go to *war* over it. But there's a good chance you've never even looked at it. At least not up-close and personal. Any guesses?!

Yes, pussy rules the world, but the crazy thing is we as women often don't see that—both literally and figuratively. In a recent survey, 48% of women said they think their vulvas are ugly and around the same amount of women have never even *looked* down there. Well, this week I'm going to reveal the secret of how to really love your pussy. It's going to send your sex life off the charts. I don't care if you've had a busload of kids; you have a thing of beauty between your legs. So over the course of the next five days, you're going to build up the boldness to really admire that million-dollar view.

This may not seem like a seduction, but it is the most important lesson in the book. I have a confession here: I'd never looked at my pussy in a mirror until I met English writer Stephanie Theobald, author of the book, *Sex Drive*. She embarks on a road trip across America looking for her lost libido. The adventure kick-starts when she meets the famous rock and roll feminist Betty Dodson, who's 90 this year. Betty has been running "masturbation master classes" for 50 years—thousands of women, from doctors and lawyers to housewives and yoga teachers, have sat naked in circles in her New York apartment and learned from this exercise.

You might be feeling a little nervous right now and if you are, well, that's why we have wine! Pour yourself a healthy glass and go get a large hand mirror. This week, your pussy gets all the attention. Every day, you're going to look (and I mean really *look*) at your pussy! You'll spend at least five minutes a day discovering the beautiful source of power, pleasure, and life between your legs.

NO. 50

#LEGENDARY

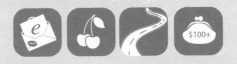

101 NIGHTS OF GREAT SEX

Now, politely ask your baby for a dinner date. If your usual Saturday night is takeout on the sofa, she'll be tickled by your invitation. And her sense of curiosity is going to get all twisted up when you explain that you will be picking her up at her friend's house. *Wait, What?!* When Saturday finally rolls around, here is precisely what the two of them will be doing all day long: *shopping*. Picking out clothes. Getting makeovers. Talking about you.

Here's what you'll do. First, a haircut—not a ten-dollar one. Find a salon where they'll give you a real once-over. They'll trim the hair off your ears and nostrils. (Yes, you have hair in both. It's gross.) One more thing: *Get your eyebrows waxed.* I'm not kidding. A decent salon will keep you looking manly but get rid of your strays.

Wash the car. Straighten up the bedroom. Put out candles. Pluck three roses' petals, sprinkle them across the bed (Make the bed first!), and put two more roses on her pillow. Time to pick her up!

Sound hard? I'll bet it's no harder than when you were courting her. That's the point. Like a true knight in shining armor, you're putting serious effort into impressing your courtly maiden. And you're going to succeed the moment she opens the door. There you are, looking better than ever, with your sharp haircut, shined shoes, best jacket, and a rose. Emotion will well up, and it will startle her to discover how much she's missed you today. This process of arriving in a clean car to pick her up feels good. It feels amazing. It feels like prom night.

Dine with her at a pretty place, in a lovely area, but don't park too close. Stroll with her. Put your arm around her, hold her hand, walk along and let her tell you about her day. Take your time; listen to what she has to say. Turn your phone to silent mode and put it away; you don't want to be checking your phone all night. On the way back to the car, find a spot under a tree and kiss her. Tell her how pretty she is, that you missed her.

When you get home, ask her to wait while you run to the bedroom. Light the candles. Tell her to come in, and just…stand there. Let her soak it in. It's an awesome sight—you, the flickering light, the roses. She might get teary; she knows you didn't have to do this. *You had her at "hello."* She's already yours, but you're putting yourself on the line like a high school crush, working your ass off, making her feel desirable, precious, loved.

You are *so* getting laid tonight. Not a gentlemanly way of looking at it, but hey, this ain't television. Here in real life, you're fixing to get some action. *Awwww.* Fade to black.

NO. 50 #LEGENDARY

INGREDIENTS

6 roses

1 good haircut

2 shined shoes

1 clean car

several candles

elbow grease

your girl's best friend

SOME SAY CHIVALRY IS DEAD. But tonight, you're bringing it back to life! Chivalrous dating habits—bringing flowers, holding hands, carrying bags—may sound quaint to a modern, split-the-check guy, but what those traits really are is *respectful*. Women on every part of the planet respond to respect—it never goes out of style. Women also respond to spontaneity, so when you surprise her with your old-fashioned chivalry, she'll undoubtedly have a huge surprise for you in return.

It's easy to make fun of old-fashioned behavior. If you spend too many nights watching 90's sitcoms on Netflix, you'll start believing the world is full of super-independent, sassy mamas who'll turn you into a punch line if you dare hold the door for them. Cue the laugh track! But that's TV. Real women love gentlemen (especially in the year 2020 when they're few and far between) and are impressed by guys who keep doing sweet, thoughtful things *even after sleeping with us*. It makes you irresistible. It makes us, um, horny.

An ultra-romantic date requires both planning and assistance—and the best place to turn for help is *your sweetheart's best friend*. Explain the following to her:

> You're planning a surprise. You need her help to get your sweetie out of the house Saturday. Your girl needs to get dressed and primped *at the friend's house*, because you're picking her up there.

Wow. All three of those things will completely impress the best friend (and make you a hero in your honey's eyes). If this were a TV sitcom, she would say *awwww,* as would the audience.

SEND HER THE TEASER!

TYPE THE LINK BELOW. CASE SENSITIVE.

101nights.com/Legendary

NO. 51

LOVE IT, RIP IT!

smooth by tight nylon. My friend Marty describes pantyhose as *giftwrap* over the sexiest present in the world. What a great image! *C'est si sexy, non?*

So…are you ready to sacrifice a good pair of pantyhose for a great lay?

Get your guy to agree to a date this weekend. On the night of the date, early in the evening, start walking around the house in an outfit that you will probably think is unfinished, and he will think is totally arousing. On top, *you're wearing a long sweater*, one that ends right at the top of your thighs. On bottom, you're wearing nothing but pantyhose. Sheer-to-the-waist pantyhose—a bit more expensive but, according to my sources, the sexiest thing on the planet. Your girly bits are mostly hidden under the sweater, but as you walk around the house, your man will quickly start to notice that you are practically naked under there. Practically, but not *quite* naked. And that is one of the sexy secrets to pantyhose.

Flirt with him. Make sure your sweater hikes up. Have him sit on the sofa while you pose for him, and dance for him. He'll be hypnotized by the sight of your bottom, your labia, your bush, all pressed together behind the barely-visible fabric. Sit on his lap and ask if he likes what you're wearing. Kiss him while he tells you how much he loves the way they fit. Ask if he wants a better look. Push him onto his back and climb up his chest. Kneel over his face. *"I was worried about wearing them in public,"* you say, *"Because you can see right through them. Can't you?"*

Kneel closer to his face. Bring your lower lips within inches of his own. Push your nylon-covered mound against his mouth, and moan. Back off, catch your breath, then push again, harder. *"Oh, that feels so good. I think you should keep that up."*

Rock your hips. Bounce a little, and let him hear the pleasure in your voice. By now, he will have noticed a flaw. There's a small hole, a rip, right on the center seam. He doesn't need to know that you put it there, hours ago, before you even pulled the stockings on. But his tongue has found it and made it obvious.

Reach down between your thighs and slip the tips of your fingernails into the hole. Tug the edges further apart, then press your unwrapped flesh even harder against his mouth. Let him hear you gasp. *"I want you in me!"* you tell him, and soon he will be, his hard shaft ripping the seam apart, the tight fabric scratching and squeezing his erection on every thrust. Your warmth and wetness is more than a gift unwrapped. For him, it's a treasure taken, a secret exposed. Tonight, you've given him so much more than sex. Your actions have validated his most secret hope: you find him so irresistible that you can't wait for intimacy. You think he is so sexy that you would rather rip your clothes than put off sex for one more second. For a man, there is no higher compliment than spontaneous sex.

Even if you had to plan it yourself.

NO. 51 LOVE IT, RIP IT!

INGREDIENTS

1 pair sheer-to-waist pantyhose, in any pattern or texture

1 pair scissors

1 thigh-length sweater

1 pair of stiletto pumps

"Men love ripping tights."

— MY FRIEND, WRITER
AND FORMER PLAYBOY
ADVISOR, ANNA DEL GAIZO

SEND HIM THE TEASER!

TYPE THE LINK BELOW. CASE SENSITIVE.

101nights.com/LoveItRipIt

ACCORDING TO *Marie Claire*, the people happiest with their sex lives live in Belgium. Belguim! That got me thinking. One reason might be that Belgians love sensual fabrics. They have a history with fabric that goes back hundreds of years; it was a giant industry for them, back in the days of the great sailing fleets. And even now they have an appreciation for luxe on a loom. They love silk, they love lace, they love…*pantyhose*.

And it turns out, so do the Royals. Those glam girls of England, Megan Markle, Kate Middleton and her younger sister, Pippa, have made pantyhose hot again. No, not the thick, matte, support hose your grandma wore. Sheer, nude and buttery, these ladies have not only made pantyhose fashionable again, but also totally sexy.

While American women have been turning their noses up at traditional hosiery for over a decade, Europeans in general (and Kate Middleton in particular) wear them often and relish showing them off. There are blogs (and yes, quite a few fetish sites) devoted to the beauty and sheer sexiness of women wearing hosiery, in every color and pattern, whole and shredded. I was especially moved by the work of famed Belgian photographer Rik Scott, and after I saw how outrageously gorgeous his models looked wearing pantyhose, the thought hit me:

I've never used pantyhose for sex. Not in my personal life, or in any of the five-hundred-plus seductions I've written. I've always been a stockings-and-garter-belt girl. I posted the pantyhose question on my my blog, and—Holy Hosiery, Batman!—the answer was a resounding yes. American men *love* the look of pantyhose!

The men I talked to told me about prom dates and secretaries, schoolteachers and MILFs, and sneaking glances up long, long legs made shiny and

NO. 52

SATIN STROKES

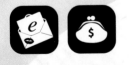

fingers is dripping with seduction. Extend your arm and drop his shirt. Hold your arm out a bit longer than necessary. Tease him as you walk around him. When his pants have dropped, lead him backwards till he is sitting on the edge of the bed with his feet planted on the floor, and stand between him and the mirror.

Now run your hands across his skin, tracing his collarbone, circling his nipples, raking your fingers up his thighs and continuing to the tip of his penis. He's going to love how cool and smooth and sensual it feels, and he's going to be *hard*. Get behind him, straddling his body with your legs. "*Look at that,*" as you snake your arms under his and stroke his hardening shaft, "*Look at us.*" Your satiny fingers on his erection and the slickness of your slip will surround him, and your whispered reminders to watch what's happening in the mirror will make him ache.

"*Would you like a happy ending?*"

Gulp.

Watch yourselves in the mirror as your hand strokes his erection. Feel how nicely the satin slides over his stiffness. Take your time and watch his face in the mirror as you stroke him, "*Mmm, I like this.*"

Here's the part where you blow his mind: Ask him to show you how he gets himself off, "*Baby, would you show me how you do it?*" Assure him that you think it's hot (*It is!*), and that you want to see what he does to make himself come.

Now, watch what he does. Let him focus on the sensation of being held by you while he masturbates. Whisper encouraging things to him, "*That looks so good...I love watching you do that...you're making me so hot.*"

Now, reach around and try your hand. Remember the speed he used, and how tightly he gripped himself. Brace yourself for his orgasm. When he seems close, whisper, "*I want you to come for me.*" When he does, catch as much as you can on your gloves. Don't forget to sneak a peek in the mirror while it's happening.

Once he's finished and his breathing's returned to normal, show him what he did to your pretty gloves. He'll love it, and wonder how he got so lucky.

Then take the gloves off, toss them aside, and give him *the look*. He may be spent, but that doesn't mean it's over. Because every girl deserves her own happy ending.

INGREDIENTS

Pair of elbow-length or opera-length gloves

satin slip dress

sexy shoes

a full-length, wardrobe mirror (available on Amazon for $19.95)

YOU'RE GOING TO RUIN a pair of gloves this week. And it's going to be *so* worth it.

I talked with a lot of people while researching this book, and while I wasn't surprised to find that massage is a popular romantic activity, I was amazed when I found out that there are places around the world where women give massages while wearing gloves. And I'm not talking about household gloves, either. Full-length, *satin opera gloves*. Wow. Now *that* is something special. *That* is something worth trying.

Gloves enhance a woman's arms, wrists and hands—some of the most expressive parts of her body. They don't *have* to be satin; there are sexy latex and leather gloves available as well, in different colors and lengths. Most adult boutiques will have something suitable, or go online to find a pair. Midweek, leave the gloves someplace he'll notice them, like draped over a chair or on top of his laptop. If he asks you what they're doing there, smile and tell him, "*They're for Saturday. For your happy ending.*" And leave it at that.

Saturday, after dinner, excuse yourself and go to the bedroom. Set a mirror about three feet from the edge of the bed and dim the lights. Step into your lingerie and shoes, and then pull the gloves on. Walk straight up to where your sweetheart is and stroke a finger under his chin in a "come hither" motion. Kiss him and say, "Follow me."

In the bedroom, *slowly* undress him in front of the mirror. As you do, exaggerate the movements of your hands. They are encased in gorgeous gloves, and every flourish you make with your wrists and

SEND HIM THE TEASER!

TYPE THE LINK BELOW. CASE SENSITIVE.

101nights.com/
SatinStrokes

NO. 53

HEELS ON A DASH

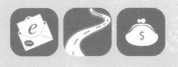

101 NIGHTS OF GREAT SEX

of all the fun you're going to be having on the way there, so make sure you set out 30 minutes early. Make sure also that you take the scenic route or the back roads, because shortly into your drive, you're going to say to her, *"You know, I'd really love you to take your panties off."*

She'll giggle at the idea, but be persistent. Don't take no for an answer. Remind her about the book! You're both reading it and this, tell her, is Seduction #53 which she's just going to LOVE. Add something like, *"Here, I'll make it easier."*

Turn up the heat in the car. Crack a window to help the hot air escape. Once she has her bare butt on the passenger seat (and isn't that something to think about next time you're driving alone?), reach over and touch her. Play with her. Dare her to put her feet up on the dash, legs splayed wide, pussy exposed. And *ohhh, that warm air, blowing up over her kitty, tickling her, warming her bottom*—it's an amazing sensation.

Tell her you have another surprise for her, waiting in the glove box. Ask her to hand it to you now. *It's her vibrator.* The sight of it alone will get her turned on even more. And the beauty of this modern wonder is that you can operate it without ever taking your eyes off the road. Just reach over and get it in the neighborhood, and the powerful buzz will find its way to her clit. You're giving her an awesome fantasy. She's exposed in public, though no one can see. She's riding a toy, but not in control. She's warm below, cool above; surrounded by rushing air and passing lights and the roar of tires and the glow of stars. She's going to come, hard.

Do you have time for a pit stop before you arrive at your final destination? Then find a dark, quiet spot and—I dare you—pull over. Pull it out. And drive it home.

NO. 53 HEELS ON A DASH

INGREDIENTS

1 car

1 vibrator

1 cool evening

1 appointment (set a little later than she thinks it is)

1 quiet dark road

How cool does it have to be before you'll turn on the car heater?

For my guy, it's *never* cold enough. I swear, there has to be frost on the windshield before he'll turn up the heat. But like most women, I love the car heater. It's toasty and warm, and the best part is that it bakes my chilly little toes first, then sends waves of warmth up my shivering legs, like I'm standing over a giant blow dryer. When I'm wearing a short skirt on a cool night, it feels great to step into that blast of heat coming up from the floorboard. It's more than relaxing; it's arousing. And this week, I want you to show your woman just how hot an evening drive can be.

Get into gear by sending her the Tease. Then, a couple of days later send her a text telling her she'll need to wear a skirt on your trip out on Saturday night. She might come back with "Why a skirt?" but you'll have piqued her curiosity. Tell her that you're taking her somewhere special. You're not going to tell her where as you want it to be a surprise.

There's a bit of trickery in setting this up. You'll need to add some extra time to your drive because

SEND HER THE TEASER!

TYPE THE LINK BELOW. CASE SENSITIVE.

101nights.com/
HeelsOnADash

NO. 54

TRIPLE THREAT

take a little extra effort to impress your honey. My recommendation: White cotton undies. White dress shirt, unbuttoned. And the pièce de résistance, *white thigh high stockings*. Ah, what a look. So pure and virginal, yet so sexy.

Secret Two: Morning Sex. Leave your guy asleep as you slip into the bathroom to put on your do-me-now white outfit. Climb back onto the bed so that you're facing him—or, more to the point, that he's facing you the moment he opens his eyes. Which he will do shortly after you lift one of your stocking-clad feet and start tickling his face with your toes. As he wakens, slide your leg down his chest. Smile, and let him admire the view.

Secret Three: The Velvet Tongue. If you haven't noticed, "The Velvet Tongue" is another seduction in the book. This is a classic. This move should be a part of every woman's bedroom repertoire. Once you have gotten a rise out of your sleeping giant, lean over to your nightstand to pick up a cup of hot tea, or coffee, or whatever. Take a sip and hold it a moment before you swallow. And now that your mouth is exceptionally hot and wet, lean over his hips, bring his shaft to your lips, and slide it in. *Ahhhhhh…* Tease him by breaking off your oral treat every minute or two, just long enough to take another steamy sip, and then bring him back to a boil.

And now that you're a Triple Threat, get even more creative. I challenge you to start customizing your own recipes for great sex. They say that women are natural multi-taskers. And we can have multi-orgasms. This week, do both. (And do it all before breakfast!)

NO. 54 TRIPLE THREAT

INGREDIENTS

1 pair white thigh-high stockings

1 pair white undies

1 white shirt

1 alarm clock

1 cup of hot tea or other hot beverage

I LOVE THE MONTHS WHEN I AM WORKING ON on a new book like this one. *Love* them! Because my personal sex life is never better. I'm doing research into sex tricks, talking to people about their favorite bedroom tips, dreaming up erotic adventures and writing them down. It's not exactly easy. But it means that I'm thinking about sex, a lot. And guess what? That automatically makes sex happen more often.

I'll bet the same thing will happen to you. As you go through this book and take on these seductions, you'll constantly be reminded how much you love the intimacy, the excitement and the pure physical fun of sex with your favorite man in the world.

So, the other day, I woke up early and horny. And I decided to try one of my, no, two of my—no wait, *three* of my favorite tricks all at once. It's a Mix 'n' Match Sale at the Corn Store! Buy one, get two free!

Secret One: Dress-Up Sex. This doesn't have to be elaborate. The reason it works is not the fancy outfit, it's the fact that you cared enough to

SEND HIM THE TEASER!

TYPE THE LINK BELOW. CASE SENSITIVE.

101nights.com/
TripleThreat

FOR **HIS EYES** ONLY

NO. **55**

HOW FAR
WILL SHE GO?

101 NIGHTS OF GREAT SEX

the Teaser to set the tone. Then a morning or two later, when you're both at work or she's off doing her own thing for the day—and you know you'll both be home alone later—start with the first text: *Hey, sexy. I want you to stop whatever you're doing right now. Go into the bathroom and send me a photo of yourself.* Surprise! This "ordinary" day is about to take a super-charged turn.

She'll probably protest a little: *You mean right now?* But she'll be smiling into her phone, guaranteed. *Yes, now. Do it,* you respond and while it may take her a few minutes, she'll oblige you. It's likely her first selfie airs on the side of innocence. Think parted plump lips, deep eye contact and some cleavage. Your response is very important! Be enthusiastic and lay it on thick: *Babe, you look so hot! You're so sexy.* Throw in a specific compliment and, if you feel like it, a flame emoji or two.

Now that you've got your banter going, it's time to get instructional with your model. She craves direction, and you're in the director's chair. She *wants* to know what you *want* to see. Moreover, women find it hot when men know and then tell you exactly what they desire. A boy asks if he can kiss you; a man just does it. The same concept applies to selfies. A boy asks for a hot photo; a man calmly commands one. Feel free to tell her where to go, how to stand or sit down and if she's home, what to wear, or not wear, for your impromptu photo shoot.

Wait a little while before the next text: *All right, goddess. Now I want you to sneak off and strip down. Show me more.* As the stakes are raised, so does the sexual suspense. She's got a new assignment and she's excited to complete it for you. About half an hour later, write another: *I need to see your gorgeous pussy. Pull your panties down and play with yourself.* The gushing fervor, and perhaps nastiness, levels of your responses should increase accordingly. *God, you're beautiful. You're making me so hard right now, I'm going to have to go to the bathroom and finish myself off. Look what you're doing to me!* Again, a protest: *No, baby, wait for me!*

And save more than enough you will. Suddenly, that once-innocuous *ding* alert is connected to the delicious prospect of sex, signaling an instant and intensifying dopamine rush from your brain directly to your pants. As the work day comes to an end and you begin to pulse with anticipation, tell your newly minted selfie queen exactly where you want her by the time you get home: *Fully naked and waiting for you in bed.* At this point, the juices, creative and otherwise, are flowing and you're about to meet your muse in real life.

Show her how much she inspires you.

HOW FAR WILL SHE GO?

INGREDIENTS

2 phones (one with a functional camera)

"One might simplify this by saying: men act and women appear. Men look at women. Women watch themselves being looked at. This determines not only most relations between men and women but also the relation of women to themselves."

-JOHN BERGER, WAYS OF SEEING

"Send nudes." Chances are you've sent this text verbatim to your lady at some point in your relationship. If you haven't blatantly thrown out the request (which these days, is the modern dating equivalent of saying, "I'm into you"), you've certainly thought it. Or perhaps you've sent out of selfie of your own in hopes of receiving an even more enticing one in return. Men love getting pics! You are visual creatures, and what kind of text is more exciting to receive than a shot of your woman, seducing you all over again from the glow of your smartphone? It's a virtual present, for your eyes and your eyes only.

I'm willing to bet she's much better at snapping scandalous selfies than you are, and that's not just because women, what with their softness and curves, tend to be easier on the eyes than their male counterparts. It's because she's practiced this; she's thought about her best angles and cutest facial expressions for years. But that doesn't mean she's a hundred-percent comfortable offering up images of herself. Sending steamy pics can be intimidating, no matter how confident you are. That's where you come in.

This seduction requires the bare minimum of planning, and that's part of the beauty of it. Send

SEND HER THE TEASER!

TYPE THE LINK BELOW. CASE SENSITIVE.

101nights.com/
HowFarWillSheGo

NO. **56**

COME CLEAN, COME DIRTY

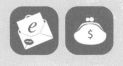

it features a hottie on a horse! Just avoid anything advertised by a football player, or sold by the quart. Do *not* use the same cologne you wore to your senior prom. The best scents can be kind of expensive, as you know if you've ever bought the real stuff at a department store. But you don't need a big bottle for this seduction—one of those little sample tubes will do. And thanks to the internet, there's a great way to get your hands on all the samples you could ever want, delivered to your door at a buck a pop. Or go to a department store and go to the cologne counter for a few free samples. A great source for this is listed in the ingredients, but the hottest scents around (according to all the surveys) are right here, under your nose:

· Dior Sauvage

· Giorgio Armani Acqua Gio Absolu

· Chanel Bleu de Chanel

· Hermès Terre d'Hermès

· Versace Eros

· Issey Miyake L'Eau d'Issey Pour Homme

· Le Labo Santal 33

· And if you insist on going old-school, try Guy Laroche Drakkar Noir

Ready? Then go ahead and slip back into bed. She's going to wake up and smell paradise.

Start easy, with lots of nuzzling and touching. If she pulls back and says something about her morning breath, reach to the nightstand for your second secret weapon: Altoids. (Did you know they're not just for blowjobs??)

Smell-Good Sex is usually *slo-oo-ow* sex, and with that luscious scent drifting from you, she's going to want to be face-to-face…or face-to-neck, and face-to-chest. Start on top, hold her close and pump away, allowing your new aroma to fuel her fantasies. Make sure she has all the orgasms she wants, because that's what will activate your third secret weapon: a scientifically-proven phenomenon called imprinting. From now on, every time she smells that fragrance on you, she's going to think of sex, and how much she wants it.

Come to think of it, maybe you should buy the bigger bottle.

NO. 56 COME CLEAN, COME DIRTY

INGREDIENTS

1 tin of Altoids or other breath mints

1 early shower

1 new cologne or aftershave (For the frugal romantic, buy cologne samples at Parfumsraffy.com)

"I can hug a man — even one I barely know, and if he smells great, I just want to f*** him!"

— MY FRIEND, STACY
(and almost the entire female population)

Bottom Line: Smell just right, and you will get laid. That's one of those universal truths, across all species. Every critter that *can* have sex, *will* have sex, if the scent checks out okay.

For most animals, of course, it's more about musk and pheromones. And butt-sniffing, if you're my dog, Sam. Sadly, though, humans don't really have a strong response to pheromones, in spite of what you read in those cheesy ads all over the internet. (Just who *is* that Dr. Athena, anyway??) Men need a little help in that department. And fortunately, there's an entire multi-billion-dollar industry standing by, just waiting to give you a hand.

The only trick to this seduction is getting out of bed a little early on Saturday morning without waking your sweetie. Jump in the shower and get squeaky clean. Make sure your mouth is sparkly fresh — use toothpaste and mouthwash. You don't really need deodorant this soon, but if you use it, pick one that's clear and unscented.

Now for your first secret weapon: a touch of cologne. A *light* touch, please. Don't splash it on; don't rub it over your face. The best way to apply it is the same way women do: Spray it into the air, wait three seconds, then walk through the mist of fragrance.

So what should you buy? Well, there's the tried and true Old Spice, which is even sexier now that

SEND HER THE TEASER!

TYPE THE LINK BELOW. CASE SENSITIVE.

101nights.com/
ComeCleanComeDirty

NO. 57

"I THINK I MADE
HIS BACK
FEEL BETTER"

BETTER"

Undress him and ask him to lie face down on the bed. Stand where he can watch while you peel down to bra and panties, then climb on top. Mmm, isn't it nice to straddle the powerful muscles in a man's back? Tension melts away as you massage warm oil into his skin. Then ask him:

Do you want to help make me come? Then I need you to stay very, very still....

Pull off your lingerie. He'll love the velvet touch of your bare breasts as you stretch out across his back. Slide your hands down his arms; braid your fingers into his own. Keep moving, keep touching. Make love to his back. Rock your hips in slow, small circles, pressing your mons directly against his tailbone. You're looking for a certain spot, a place that's just right for your clitoris to snuggle in to. You'll know when you find it!

Now you can stoke your own fire. Let your aching clit set the pace as it rubs against his oil-soaked skin, up and down and around. When you find that special place, that groove — then start moving faster. He can't see you, so let your fantasies run wild. And let him know what's happening...whisper in his ear that you're getting close, and closer. Pinch his nipples, suck his neck. Hold him tight! Let him feel every twitch of your orgasm.

After all, you've become the bedmate men dream of — a woman who can get all the foreplay she wants...

All by herself!

INGREDIENTS

1 very still man

1 bottle of oil

1 very active woman

1 mirror (optional)

SPECIAL NOTE:
For an amazing visual impact – prop a mirror up against the wall so he can watch.

"I think I made his back feel better."

MARILYN MONROE
after a private meeting with JFK

This particular seduction has such a special meaning to me. This is the trick Marilyn Monroe was famous for. More to the point, it's the technique that gave me my very first orgasm with a man.

It wasn't the first orgasm of my life. I had long ago learned the pleasure of masturbation, the same way 75 percent of women do. We become sexually stimulated by simply rubbing up against something — a pillow, perhaps a big stuffed toy, but usually nothing more than our bedsheets.

You and your lover are going to add this technique to your sexual repertoire, and along the way, he's going to discover that, like Marilyn Monroe herself, you've become every man's erotic ideal. Here's how…

SEND HIM THE TEASER!

TYPE THE LINK BELOW. CASE SENSITIVE.

101nights.com/
HisBackFeelsBetter

NO. 58

HAVANA NIRVANA

big gold or silver hoop earrings. (Did you know that according to studies, men find earrings to be the sexiest kind of jewelry?) Slide on some tiny metal bangles–the ones that jingle when they fall together. Tonight, you're not afraid to make some noise.

To set the mood, put on your playlist and turn up the thermostat. This is a night in Havana, baby, and Havana is *muy caliente*. Mix a couple of *Cuba Libres* (That's Rum and Coke!) have your guy sit in a chair, and start moving your hips to the beat. He doesn't care if you're dancing authentic Salsa Cubana or the Electric Slide; you're shaking your assets for him, and that's turning him on.

Tell him to undress while you watch, and then to lie on the bed. Strip slowly, taking off everything except for your jewelry. Crawl up his body toward his face, your nipples grazing his skin. Straddle his head and lower yourself to his mouth. Close enough so your lips touch, but not too close. "Kiss me here." Keep your clitoris just in front of his tongue. "That's it, that's so good…" Focus on moving only your hips until he's squirming beneath you.

Sweating yet? You *should* be. Your skin should be slick and dewy. Slide your body toward his *chile*. Stay there, rubbing your wetness into his shaft. Lean forward like a jockey and slide onto him. Hold very still and tense your vaginal muscles around his penis ten times slowly, then ten times quickly. Watch his look of surprise when you do—he's putty in your hands.

Sit up, move your hips in time with the music. I can't stress enough how important a good soundtrack is here! It's what takes it from warm to super-hot. Dancing all over his tongue (and pene) requires the right rhythms. Don't worry about sliding up and down yet; the sensation of your tight wetness pulling him in all directions will amaze him. Raise your arms over your head as you ride him so the bracelets fall together and jingle.

Whatever you do, don't let him finish. The role of *jinetera* is to keep the *bestia* under her control. When his body signals that he's close, lift yourself off quickly and continue your dance on his tongue. Make your way from his tongue down to his shaft and back up again at least three times. It's a real workout, but it's worth every sizzling second. You can control every inch of him with your hips and your PC muscles.

Remember, you're in charge. Don't stop teasing him until he's shaking with the effort of holding back. Finally, tell him you want him to come. Keep your eyes locked on his and never let up your grip on his shaft.

He'll wonder how sex so wild could leave him feeling so tame.

INGREDIENTS

tight-fitting outfit

pair of heels

several skinny metal bracelets

large gold hoop earrings

Salsa music

CUBAN HIPS DON'T LIE.

In a country where the average salary is $750 a month and a pair of jeans costs $80, Cuban women make do with what they have. And what they have is one hell of a sexy attitude. Tonight, you'll be taking on the role of a Cuban seductress and riding your man like a beast.

If there's one thing Cubans share, it's a love of Salsa—a huge part of Cuban culture. Thanks to Salsa, Cuban girls know how to move their hips, and grow up knowing how to drive a man wild, sexually. That's exactly what you'll do when you ride your lover like you're breaking in a wild horse.

With your hips and pelvic muscles, you'll conquer your man with a seductive dance. Start by sending him the Tease, and follow it up later with some texts. In Spanish. They'll throw him off and if he's not bilingual, he'll probably have to look them up, but that's part of the seduction. He'll instantly know things are about to get caliente. Then create your playlist: Think a great mix of classic Salsa and Cubano-inspired hits, from Buena Vista Social Club to Camila Cabello (yes, that would be "*Havana, ooh-na-na!*").

Leave the PTA skirts in the closet. Squeeze into a miniskirt or short-shorts, a halter top with plenty of cleavage, and high heels. It's about looking sexy, not perfect. Do you have belly rolls? Yeah, well, most of us do. Cuban women know that every size and shape is sexy.

Flaunt it. Walk in front of your mirror: shoulders back, ass out, hips *working* it. The more confident you are, the sexier you seem.

Tonight, you sparkle. Use shimmering body oil. And since Cuban women are conscious of their sex appeal 24/7, adorn your body with jewelry. Wear

SEND HIM THE TEASER!

TYPE THE LINK BELOW. CASE SENSITIVE.

101nights.com/ HavanaNirvana

NO. 59

INTO THE DARK

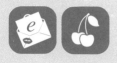

of clothing.

Here is where the magic begins. It's not the stripping that gets to her. *It's the whisper.* The heat of your breath, the tickle of sound, the surprise of your skin so close to hers. It will send a tingle down her spine. After she's pulled off the first bit of clothing, blow out one candle and leave the room. A minute later, sneak up again and seductively murmur the same order in her other ear. It doesn't seem like much, does it? But with each step you're heightening her senses, lifting her out of the realm of the ordinary. As before, blow out another candle, and disappear for a minute or two. Each time you approach her, make sure you stay behind her, so that your voice and position are always mysterious, unpredictable. Startle her with a sweet treat you know she likes, a piece of chocolate perhaps, brushed against her lips. Let her take a lick. Then with another irresistible whisper, ask her to remove one more piece of clothing. When she's done, blow out a third candle.

Now begin to touch her, but only on her back and neck. Gentle strokes, soft kisses. You're focusing attention away from the *usual* erogenous zones on the front of her body, and making every part of her yearn for a caress. Again, blow out a candle and disappear after she pulls off the next-to-last item. When you return, deliver another delicious taste to her mouth. Stay behind her, but let your hands explore more. Run your fingertips down her arms, then glide them back up to her shoulders. Slowly drop your hands down to her breasts. Drag your fingertips along the tops of her thighs. Kneel between her legs and give her one long, languorous kiss right on her lower lips. Her mind is hypnotized now by the slow rhythm of your comings and goings, the erotic touches, the darkening room. She has one last item to strip off, and you have one last candle to extinguish. One more minute to make her wait. She can hardly stand it anymore. Her nerves are buzzing, begging for more.

When you come back this last time, whisper one last sexy order.

I'm going to make love to you now. Get down on your hands and knees. That's all she needs to hear. Your magic spell is complete. She has been bewitched out of her regular life and taken to a place of enchantment; a world where she is ready for anything, ready to forget any insecurities and inhibitions, ready to take whatever you can give her, right there on her knees in the dark.

INGREDIENTS

1 small chair

5 candles

1 sheet of paper

1 or 2 sweet treats (candy, fruit, chocolate)

THERE'S A SECRET THAT ALL MAGICIANS KNOW. The human mind can be steered. With the lightest of touches, the smallest of hints and the subtlest shift in light, a good magician can direct your thoughts. They can enhance your senses, or block them; they can make you see and feel things that aren't even there. They can spin a fantasy and make you live it.

One of my favorite fantasy spinners is Michael Carbonaro of the popular show "The Carbonaro Effect." I just love him because he makes every trick look so easy, and as it turns out, some of them are! It simply takes the right kind of man to execute an illusion, and this week *you're* that man. After all, who doesn't want to learn a good magic trick. Especially if it involves sex.

This week I challenge you to use a little trickery to help your lover hit new highs. All you need for this performance is a chair, five candles, and a cryptic text message saying: *Bedroom, 7pm. Wear only five articles of clothing.* If she comes back with a "Why five?" be firm. Tell her, *"Five is the magic number. Wear six and you'll be punished."*

Already, she's mystified, and that's the first step in any magic trick. That night she'll enter the room at seven to see all five candles burning, and the chair placed in the middle of the floor. Tell her to sit, eyes closed, facing away from the door. Now make her wait. Just for a minute or two. Let her sense of anticipation build. Then, as quietly as you can, sneak up behind her, bring your lips close to her ear, and in a whisper, tell her to remove one item

SEND HER
THE TEASER!

TYPE THE LINK BELOW. CASE SENSITIVE.

101nights.com/
IntoTheDark

NO. 60

BALLERS CLUB

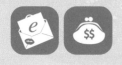

When she sees that you've scattered the bed with even more dollar bills, she'll be nodding like crazy. But you're not going to let her have it just yet. Your conversation might go something like this:

Where did you find all that money?

"Around the house"

You didn't earn it, did you?

"No"

Well, now you're going to earn it

The Ballers Club tends to takes on a life of its own. Some of you will want to play out the whole nasty fantasy: You're the high roller who just won $6 million at Blackjack and you've come to claim the top escort girl in Sin City. If your gal's anything like me, she'll have a secret fantasy about being paid to have sex. And now that you're dressed up like Dwayne Johnson and projecting movie star confidence, she's going to want to get going.

And for those of you not into role play, this is going to be a super-passionate night because, guess what? A bed full of crisp dollar bills simply calls out for some hot doggy style! After some heavy kissing and sexy banter (you *did* just make it rain!), instruct her to get on all fours, then kneel behind her and smooth some of those dollar bills in her panties into her clit. Whisper into her ear, "Do you like money?" She'll start to moan that she actually *loves* money, especially when she feels your hard cock pushing from behind against her butt cheeks.

She'll be soaking at this point, but you're going to say, "I don't think you like money enough yet." Take her panties and bra off and push her gently down into the bed so she's rubbing her whole naked body over that sexy pile of bills. This will be thrilling for her; it's unlikely she's ever done this before. It's the sort of thing good girls don't do and she'll love it for that very reason.

When the time's right, tell her to get up on all fours again. Take a handful of dollars and rub them over her breasts and erect nipples as you rub your penis between her legs and on her clit. Get her really warmed up before you penetrate her. By now she's got dollar signs in her eyes and affirmative moans coming from her lips.

Now you're going to go in, and you're going to love the ride. Imagine you're the high roller who just $20 million at the tables and this lady you're pumping is the golden prize. Nothing turns a woman on more than power, and as she gazes at the faces of scores of George Washingtons lying there on the mattress as her hunky man does her from behind, she's on for one of the most unforgettable orgasms of her life. Don't be surprised if she screams, "Yes! I love money! I love *you*!" as you both shudder to an intense climax.

Welcome to the Ballers Club!

INGREDIENTS

$60-$500 in dollar bills

One well-tailored suit

One confident,
high-rolling guy

THERE'S NOT A GUY WHO DOESN'T LOOK GREAT holding a big wad of money, and this week, that guy's going to be YOU.

You've heard of a roll around in the hay? Well, the Ballers Club takes things to a whole new level, because smelling money is way sexier than smelling straw!

Start by sending the Tease, which will automatically let her know you've got something fun in store. Next, at least a few hours later, a text: *You're going to be finding some precious pieces of paper this week. Grab them up and wait until I tell you what's next.* Remember, this seduction is about you calling the shots. Money is power, right?

Then, throughout the week, you're going to be creating a treasure hunt of dollar bills around the house. Leave them in her shoes, in her make-up bag, leave a little trail of them by the chair she sits in to watch TV. Your budget can be anything from $60 to $500. The more dollar bills, the better you're going to look, obviously, although whatever the amount, she's going to be totally intrigued, thinking, *Oh my god, I keep finding dollar bills every day! Whaaat is he doing?!*

On the big day, send another text announcing you're happy to confirm she is eligible for membership to the exclusive Ballers Club. Tell her she needs to knock on the bedroom door at a specified time wearing all those dollar bills tucked into her sexiest lingerie.

Once she gets to the bedroom, she'll be raring to go. She's got a stack of money rubbing against her nipples and her clit and she's dying to know what happens next. And when she sees you standing there, looking like the Cincinnati Kid in your best suit and holding a handful of yet more bills, she's going to think her birthday came early.

Enjoy watching her standing there with all that money in her panties and bra and then say, "Good evening and welcome to the Ballers Club. Are you ready for your initiation?"

SEND HER THE TEASER!

TYPE THE LINK BELOW. CASE SENSITIVE.

101nights.com/BallersClub

NO. 61

POWER STRIP

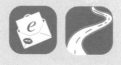

grocery store? Now take your shirt off, and grab a broom. Take a photo of yourself grinning and sweeping the floor, then send it to her. Get out your toolbox and snap a shot of you with your cordless screwdriver. She'll look forward to each new *ding* on her phone, waiting to see what surprises you've been cooking up. Ooh, cooking! Now there's a chore she'd like to see you perform! Send a picture of you in your undies and an apron. And then another with you wearing an apron *and nothing else*. Shot from behind.

Next photo: you with a tool belt and a smile. Next: Rubber gloves. Monkey wrench. Vacuum cleaner. Take a series of selfies, each time doing a different chore, and each time getting more and more naked. Send them to her phone, one at a time. Include an occasional text message:

> *Can't wait to see you.*
>
> *Working hard.*
>
> *Ready to play.*
>
> *Like what you see?*
>
> *Come home soon.*

Of course, you must complete at least one real chore, like cleaning the windows. Remember, it's *actual work* that gets her hot. The sight of your bare buns will make her laugh. (Especially if she sees them while she's in a grocery store!) But the thought of you naked *while* relieving her of housework is what makes her tingle.

As soon as she gets home, put some britches on, because you need to help her put away the groceries. Then repeat your striptease, live and in person.

And then get to work. On *her*.

no. 61 POWER STRIP

INGREDIENTS

2 smartphones

household cleaning supplies

big smile

clean underwear

WHEN IT COMES TO AROUSING A WOMAN, timing is everything. Usually, that means making sure she is relaxed and not facing any distractions.

But this week, it means you have to wait…until she's at the grocery store. No, seriously.

Right after she leaves for a weekend grocery run, you are going to begin doing the one thing that makes all women melt: *chores*. Household chores. Cleaning, fixing, straightening. Most men instinctively avoid housework, but that's only because they don't realize how much it turns women on. Those reality home makeover shows, where crews of men come in and fix everything that's wrong with your house? That's *girl porn*. Pure erotica.

Are you still reading? Good. I was afraid I might have scared you away with the chores idea. You won't actually have to work hard this week. You just have to give the appearance of housework— and combine it with the appearance of stripping. *And* catch it all on camera.

Begin with some glass cleaner and paper towels. Take a selfie of you wiping down a window and send it to your sweetie.. What do you suppose the other shoppers will make of it when they hear her crack up laughing in the middle of the

SEND HER THE TEASER!

TYPE THE LINK BELOW. CASE SENSITIVE.

101nights.com/PowerStrip

FOR **HIS EYES** ONLY

NO. 62

BONE APPÉTIT

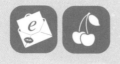

101 NIGHTS OF GREAT SEX

Preparation is easy. Dinner can be takeout from your favorite restaurant. Just dress it up a little by serving it on real plates with a couple of candles. By the time she gets out of the bathroom—clean, smelling great, wearing a cute skirt and a grin from ear-to-ear—she's going to be the happiest woman in town. Enjoy your meal. Have a drink. Or two.

Then whip out the handcuffs.

What, no cuffs in your toolbox?? Then buy a pair! Before your sweetie gets up from the table, give her a big kiss...let her see your new toy and play with it for a moment...and then gently lock her wrists together behind the chair.

Kneel in front of her. Slide your hand between her knees and move them apart, hiking her skirt up as you go. Kiss her thighs and her hips. Nibble at the edge of her undies...nibble her through her undies...and then tug them aside. She can't help, she can't stop, she can't do anything at all right now except enjoy being the focus of your attention and your love. And your tongue. Remind her that, of all those 30,000-plus meals you've had in your life, she's still your favorite thing to eat...

You're not quite done yet, though. To make this truly a meal for the ages, a dinner that glows forever in her memory, you still have to do two remarkable, wonderful things:

1) Bring her to a shuddering climax.

And then:

2) Do the dishes.

NO.62 BONE APPÉTIT

INGREDIENTS

1 pair of handcuffs

1 bath

candles

dinner with light appetizers or salads

babysitter as needed

THREE MEALS A DAY, SEVEN DAYS A WEEK. By the time you're 28 years old, you've eaten more than 30,000 meals. But how many do you actually remember? How many are so special that you talk about them years later? Here's one that will go right to the top of that list, a dinner you'll never forget. Or, to be more precise, a dinner your woman will never forget.

Start by letting her know that you're taking charge. Early in the week, send her a text like this one.

> *You are going to LOVE Saturday night. Kids will be at your mom's—I'll have dinner ready at seven. You don't even have to dress up because we're staying home. But a skirt would be nice. Yes, a skirt would be perfect. Wear a skirt. ;-)*

Dinner, no kids and *you're taking care of everything*?? Oh, she is so looking forward to the weekend now. But just to keep her on the edge of anticipation, send one more text on Friday:

> *Did I mention you should wear a skirt tomorrow night?   Love - Me*

SEND HER THE TEASER!

TYPE THE LINK BELOW. CASE SENSITIVE.

101nights.com/ BoneAppetit

NO. 63

A DARING
DESSERT

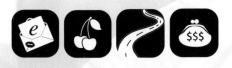

perform a tease-filled twist on every man's fantasy: you'll be practically naked in the restaurant, but he'll be the only one who knows it.

At the end of the meal, excuse yourself to the restroom (take your coat). Inside the restroom, shed your dress and slip on the coat. When you come back to the table, hand him your dress, as nonchalantly as if you're giving him a napkin. There may be a moment of confusion for him. But watch his face as the realization dawns on him that *you're almost naked*, right there, in the middle of the restaurant, and you've done it all to stoke the fire of his dirty little mind.

As you slide back into your seat, tell him that you heard about a delectable dessert not listed on the menu. Let him know how hot you are, that you're just dying to take off that suffocating coat, by sticking one leg out toward him as far as you dare, and running your foot up his leg. Tell him you want him to take you to the coatroom, the bathroom, or the parking lot (*anywhere!*) and help you out of your coat like a true gentleman. Flash him just a peek at what you've got (or haven't got) on underneath.

You'll never hear a faster "Check please!" in your life!

NO. 63 A DARING DESSERT

INGREDIENTS

daring lingerie

1 dress

1 trenchcoat

1 confident woman

1 trendy restaurant

SOME FOODS IGNITE SEXUAL DESIRE, and wine never fails to set an amorous mood. But tonight what's on the table will merely be a side dish. The main course is *you*.

Make dinner reservations at your favorite dark, romantic restaurant. Put on that hot little thing you know drives him wild, whether it's a garter belt with seamed stockings or a bustier with a thong. Then top that off with a dress that won't give away what lies beneath. For your final layer, don a long coat.

Take your man out for a dinnertime surprise. Eat well, give him flirtatious looks, rub his calves with your foot. Feed him little bites off your fork and exchange kisses across the table.

He'll think that's all pretty amazing, but wait until you get to the true chef's special: You're going to

SEND HIM
THE TEASER!

TYPE THE LINK BELOW. CASE SENSITIVE.

101nights.com/
ADaringDessert

FOR **HIS EYES** ONLY

NO. **64**

WICKED VIEW

101 NIGHTS OF GREAT SEX

sensitive, private part right under the flow. Tease her with your hand; slide your fingers into those delicious, sensitive folds of flesh, and finally open her lips wide to the coursing water.

She'll be excited and more than a little surprised—surprised that you know this trick (although many women do!), shocked that she is essentially masturbating right in front of you.

And now you're going to blow her away.

Pile up some of those big towels in the tub as a cushion for her head and shoulders —and your knees. Slip off your robe, straddle her in the tub and kneel right above her face...but don't let her take you in her mouth. Instead, stroke yourself. Make yourself hard. Show her, up close and very personal, just how you like to be touched.

Chances are she's never watched a man play with himself like this before. The fact that you're standing above her, stroking your cock because that's how much she turns you on is sexy in itself. But the fact that you didn't ask permission or second-guess yourself, that's what takes it to new levels. Ballsy? In more ways than one! It's a confident move, one she'll find herself fantasizing about for months to come.

She's also never had quite this much warm, gushing, constant stimulation to her swollen clitoris before. The combination will send her out of control, beyond her usual limits, and headed for one of the greatest orgasms of her life—one that you gave her, and one she'll never forget.

NO.64 WICKED VIEW

INGREDIENTS

2 candles

1 robe

music

silky bath oil

lots of towels

1 spotless bathtub

THE GREATEST ORGASMS HAPPEN when we try something new—something that startles us and surprises us and drives us way over our sexual speed limits. Tonight, you're going to give your lover one of those landmark orgasms.

Tonight, you're going to push her right over the edge.

Start by turning your bathroom into a palace of pleasure for your mistress. Candlelight, scented bath oil, mounds of big fluffy towels and her favorite music playing on Spotify. Lead her to the tub and help her in; sit on the edge and spend lots of time washing and caressing her. Her mind will relax as her skin comes alive; she'll probably assume that this royal treatment is the whole seduction—*Ahhh*, but she'll be wrong.

Don't rinse her off yet. Simply start to drain the tub and tell her you want to try something new. Ask her to slide down toward the spigot...and have her spread her legs under the faucet, feet up on the wall. Adjust the flow of water carefully—not too hot! Not too hard!—and have her slip that most

SEND HER THE TEASER!

TYPE THE LINK BELOW. CASE SENSITIVE.

101nights.com/
WickedView

NO. 65

LAZY BOY, BUSY GIRL

She might be nervous, but she's more excited than anything. Explain that you have a plan to break in your newest gadget.

Place some pillows on the floor so that she's comfortable sitting down, with her back propped up against the sofa. I can't tell you the exact angle or height, since so much depends on you. Or more specifically, your anatomy. Because here's what you're going to do:

Straddle her face, knees on either side of her head, facing the sofa. Don't sit on her, or apply any pressure at all. You may have to adjust those pillows, but when you have it right, she'll be relaxed, comfortable, and staring at Mr. Friendly dangling right in front of her. You'll be at ease, too, leaning forward on the sofa for support. Hand her the vibe and say, "I want to feel you come while I'm in your mouth. Just concentrate on making yourself feel good."

Here's where things get intense. Way intense, way fast. Because for her, it's not just the vibrator. It's the huge erection filling her mouth, plus that incredibly hot dirty-girl feeling of masturbating right in front of you. For you, it's not just the sucking…as if that weren't enough. No, you also get that sense of control, that dominant take-it-in-your-mouth feeling, plus an awesome, over-the-top view: the image of your woman's face as she climaxes while clinging to your erection.

It's like having your own personal porn star, right between your legs.

NO.65 LAZY BOY, BUSY GIRL

INGREDIENTS

1 new vibrator
(something girly, like a
Lipstick Vibrator)

batteries

several pillows

HEAD'S UP

How many vibrators does she own? Well, whatever it is, it's not enough. A girl can never have too many. You can also use the "Lipstick Vibe" for seductions Tongue & Cheek and Heels on a Dash.

NO LESSON THIS TIME. No deep insight. Hey, sometimes the best thing you can do for a relationship is just to make each other come as hard as you possibly can.

And fortunately, that's easier than ever. Motors are quieter. Batteries are stronger. Charges last longer. This is the freaking Golden Age of vibrators, my friend. We live in wonderful times.

Just for fun, pick up a new vibe this week. Have it gift wrapped and then leave it conspicuously in the middle of the coffee table. Don't let her open it just yet. Let it sit there for a few days. The night before your sex date, send her the Tease, so by the time the moment rolls around she's good and warmed up.

When your girl meets you in the living room, make her wait for her surprise. There's magic in anticipation: Women can get turned on just by thinking about sex. Make out, drink wine, make out some more, and then—finally—offer to satisfy her curiosity. Smile and then let her open her gift.

SEND HER THE TEASER!

TYPE THE LINK BELOW. CASE SENSITIVE.

101nights.com/
LazyBoyBusyGirl

NO. 66

THE WETTER, THE BETTER

breast. It barely conceals the nipple. It says, "I'm almost naked." It's the good kind of trashy. If you don't have one, go buy one today.

The hardest part of your seduction is getting up a little early without waking your man. Quietly sneak out of bed, go brush your teeth, climb in the shower, and wash with one of those wonderful scented shower gels. My pick? *Green Tea*, by Estee Lauder. Yummy. The fragrance will stay with you all morning. When you step out of the shower...put on your t-shirt. Yes, I mean while you're still wet. Damp-dry your hair, and wipe off the rest of your exposed skin, but let that sheer moist cotton cling to you. In fact, splash a little more water right over your nipples. Let them peek through that sheer wet fabric.

Now go and quietly rouse your guy from his sleep. One look at you and that shouldn't be hard to do. Roll him on his back and climb on top of him, in all your glistening dream-girl glory. You may be thinking, "*Make-up! I need make-up! I need to dry my hair!*" But trust me — he's thinking "*Boobies! Wet boobies! Shiny, wet woman is giving me an erection! I've died and gone to Hooters!*" He's also probably loving the fact that you're all-natural.

The lingerie business is a multi-million dollar industry and for good reason-- there's nothing like a beautiful ensemble to make you feel sexy. But look how sexy your man thought you were in the simplest shirt on Earth. I've created a lot of seductions over the years that required some help from Victoria's Secret (or Agent Provocateur). But I think this is the first time I ever had an orgasm courtesy of good ole cotton. I guess it really is the fabric of our lives!

INGREDIENTS

scented shower gel
(Green Tea, by Estee Lauder
is a delicious option,
available on Amazon)

1 "wife-beater" t-shirt (or
tank top)

SHOWER SCENES IN MOVIES. Wet t-shirt contests in bars. Beer commercials. "Girls Gone Wild." Olympic beach volleyball. Everywhere you look, all around the world, there's a universal image that every man finds arousing: the wet woman.

Doesn't matter if she's under water, dripping wet, or just a little damp with perspiration. It looks *hot*. Men love it. And this week you're going to surprise your man with a little glistening skin in the most unlikely place.

Preparation for this seduction couldn't be easier. Everything you need is probably already in your house, except for one simple, inexpensive ingredient. It's a man's classic white undershirt, the kind with no sleeves or collar. You know it as a "wife-beater." One of your tank tops will work in a pinch.

This undershirt either looks totally great on a guy, or totally dorky. It all depends on how much time he spends at the gym. But every woman looks sexy wearing one of these t-shirts. Thin and ribbed, it reveals that lovely curve along the outside of the

SEND HIM
THE TEASER!

TYPE THE LINK BELOW. CASE SENSITIVE.

101nights.com/
TheWetterTheBetter

NO. 67

LOLA

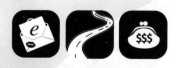

(But then again, why not?) A tailored suit with a barely visible bra peeking out can be startlingly seductive, and a short leather skirt with high heels just might steal his breath away. The object, of course, is to meet the man of your dreams for the first time—*again*.

When you arrive all alone at the bar you'll be feeling nervous but – jackpot! That's exactly what you should be feeling. Remember all those times in the past when you've pushed yourself through the fear and come out the other side feeling ecstatic? Nothing ventured, nothing gained, as they say. And your gain tonight is going to be the thrilling new you that gets created whenever you role play — and the rapt attention you're going to get from your mystery man.

You'll spot him first—remember, he's looking for the *old* you. Send him a drink, and just as the waiter points out the beautiful woman who ordered it, stroll over and introduce yourself. "Hi, I'm Lola. I'm stuck here all by myself and couldn't help notice that you seem to be in the same boat. I hope you don't mind me being so presumptuous…"

Mind?! This man is going to be thrilled by the game you're playing. You're intriguing, sexy, flirty, playful. *"Well, I'm here for the bar association meeting — did I tell you I'm an attorney? Mergers and acquisitions. And you? Oh, really, that's so interesting…"* He's witty and clever, and so obviously turned on by you. He'll start to get into the role play thing too: *"Yeah, I did the structural design work for this hotel. Turned out well; the company has me starting a new one in Honolulu next month. You know, I can't believe a woman as lovely as you isn't spoken for yet…"*

Play it up, Lola. There's something so exciting about being in a strange, glamorous bar: the smell of the leather, the sparkle of the lights, the intriguing people around you. You're creating electricity and he's seeing you as a fresh, sexy stranger who's up for some good times. There are so many 'What ifs' going on right now: Will he kiss you daringly on your naked shoulder? Will this turn into a one night stand?

The night is young, so order another round of drinks and you'll soon be feeling warm and loose and Lola will be in the mood to start whispering secrets about her other life as a showgirl in Paris. *"And do you know what used to happen after midnight when we got summoned to the count's château?"* Be prepared to be summoned to the best room in the Westin.

NO.67 LOLA

INGREDIENTS

1 fun wig

1 hotel bar

1 wickedly sexy outfit

a little perfume

1 sassy attitude

SEND HIM
THE TEASER!

TYPE THE LINK BELOW. CASE SENSITIVE.
101nights.com/Lola

"I'm in the mood for love," YOUR TEXT READS. *"So meet me tonight at eight in the lobby bar at the Westin. My name is Lola. What's yours? P.S. dress sharp!"*

You should fire off this exceptionally provocative note to your sweetie on Friday morning. You can bet his usual expression will be changed to a sly grin all day at work! Your change will be even more dramatic, though, as you're going to transform yourself into *someone else*—someone just as sweet and sharp as you, but who looks a little different, a bit more exotic. Basically, you're going to be turning yourself into a woman who's never met the hot guy who's turning up tonight in the most elegant bar in town.

My suggestion is to start by buying a wig. You've probably noticed that wigs are back in style, from candy-pink to baby blue and for a minimal amount, a hairdresser will help you put it on and make it look good. And don't forget your nails. If you normally wear red polish, then do *blue*. Or wear them long—a set of gel-coated acrylics will cost you around $50. You can really have fun with this: How about some nails with diamond studs or crystals and stars?

Why? Well, partly because romance is about the constant renewal of your relationship. Partly to remind yourselves of all the excitement and air of mystery that surrounded your first meeting. But mostly because it's *so much fun*!

Just like the hair switch, pick an outfit that's not *you*! I don't necessarily mean skimpy and sultry.

NO.**68**

STRAIGHT FLUSH

to explore.) When enacted with a trusted lover, bondage is a smoking-hot fantasy, and it is especially powerful for women—again, in that Dark Side sort of way—because it allows a good girl to give in. It gives us permission to be bad. It doesn't exactly silence that little voice in our heads that says *You're not supposed to do nasty things, but it sure does say Hey, little voice, shut up!* Whew. That's a lot of psychology for ten bucks worth of rope and a few Boy Scout knots.

And for this erotic encounter, a little tie-me-up fun is just the warm-up for your next trick. This one is a variant on another girl-fantasy classic: sex with the possibility of getting *caught*. Why do some women get so turned by that? It starts in the same place: we're taught from a young age to be good little girls, and so doing it in semi-public is just our libido's way of giving the finger to The Man. So how do you go from bound-and-pounded to almost getting caught by someone else? Here's how:

Just before she hits a climax, stop. Pick up the telephone. Start dialing. Hold the phone between you so that you can both hear what's happening on the line. At this point she will start saying something like "*Wha-a-aa, wha, what are you doing?!*" And you explain:

You are wondering (ring, ring) just how long she can keep a straight face (ring, ring) while she is talking to ("Hello?")...her best friend!

Now put the phone on the pillow right next to her head. She'll squirm. She'll mouth a silent *NO!* She will certainly blush. But her friend will say hello again, and your sweetie will have to say hi. And if not, then you take the phone and say hi. Chat for a second, and then say that your baby wanted to say hi, too. Now put the phone by her ear, and at that point what can she do but start talking to her girlfriend and pretending that nothing odd is going on—certainly nothing sexual, oh no. No ropes tying me up with my guy going down on me while we're talking, of course not, and how are you?

Now comes the next trick. Whisper in her other ear, "*Ten minutes. I dare you not to come.*" And then go back to work giving her all the pleasure you can, while she is helpless to resist, straining to keep her voice from giving anything way. All that squirming, lip-biting, inevitable giggling that comes with the mere prospect of getting caught in the act (and experiencing a deliciously uncomfortable phone call) is enough to push her over the orgasmic edge.

NO.68 STRAIGHT FLUSH

INGREDIENTS

1 phone

several feet of soft nylon rope (or 4 straps and restraint cuffs, available online or in adult boutiques everywhere)

1 bff, friend, or family member

HELPFUL HINT:
Have backup phone numbers ready. If her best friend does not answer, try her second-best friend, or her sister. Or your best friend.

SEND HER THE TEASER!

TYPE THE LINK BELOW. CASE SENSITIVE.

101nights.com/
StraightFlush

LET ME JUST MAKE IT CLEAR RIGHT UP FRONT: *sex is good.* Sex is *always* good. But sex is better when it's amplified by fantasy, no? Fantasy sex is cranked up even higher when it's propelled by certain elements we wouldn't want to discuss with, say, our mothers or ministers. Let's call that the Dark Side.

This week, you're going to use one hot fantasy for the sole purpose of sparking up another one. You're going to play with your lover's head, as well as the usual parts.

You're going to free her mind and inhibitions by taking away her power to say no.

And you're going to have a big laugh while doing it. I promise you!

Here's another trick for making good sex better. *Tease your partner.* Let her know in advance that you have something special planned. Nothing makes a pussy tingle like a little anticipation, let me tell you. So get your sweetie's morning off to an intriguing start by telling her you have a surprise for her tonight. A new little game to play. Tell her she'll know it when it happens.

Later, bring her to the bedroom and start fooling around. Get her all happy and naked and then spring your surprise—or what she *thinks* is your surprise. Under the bed you have hidden some long, soft nylon ropes, attached at one end to the legs of the bedframe. (Cool option: buy some soft Velcro cuffs and adjustable restraint straps! Professional sex paraphernalia shows you mean *business*, and only enhances the fantasy she is about

NO. 69

VIVA LA JUICY

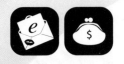

101 NIGHTS OF GREAT SEX

although knee-high ones are cute, too.

Your new thigh high tube socks will be the centerpiece of a supersexy look. Think good girl gone bad: short skirt (pleated maybe), sheer bra. White tube socks with those signature three stripes. And—do I even need to say it?—*no underwear*.

Now here comes the fun part. Call your honey into the room and let him get a good look at you. You're sitting in a chair, feet pulled up on the seat in front of you, knees up against your chest. Between your feet (and right in front of your skirt) is a small pillow. Give him a moment to admire the view. Then smile a wicked grin... and toss the pillow down on the floor in front of you. *Oh, yes.* No panties. The view just got much better.

Point to the pillow. Then to his knees. Then back to the pillow. You don't really have to say a word, do you? Once he's kneeling before you, take his head in your hands and guide him straight to your sweet spot. That's right; take control and make him do it. He loves being shown exactly how to please you. Your moans and thrusts will drive him wild. Grab his hair and push his mouth right up against you; make him lap it up for as long as you want.

Oh, he's going to get his reward tonight, you'll see to that.

But for now, all you need to do is let him enjoy the feel of those soft, sexy cotton tube socks...against the back of his neck.

NO.69 VIVA LA JUICY

INGREDIENTS

pair of thigh high tube socks (you can find them on Google)

1 pillow

1 chair

1 bra

1 skirt

TUBE SOCKS. *Tube socks!* Who would have believed that those could ever come back in style? Part of every gym class uniform in the seventies, they were laughable by the eighties and dead and buried by the nineties, alongside headbands, leg warmers, and acid-washed jeans.

But suddenly cotton socks are experiencing a comeback. Skaters and athletes and cheerleaders wear them. Models and actresses, and pop stars wear them. When I saw them all over Instagram in 2019, I knew their time had come back around again.

Old-school tall athletic socks are sexy, in a way they never were the first time around. And it's not just women who think so: There's something innocent and youthful about clean white socks that really get guys going.

In this case, the higher, the better: A pair of thigh-high tube socks that go almost all the way up to that adorable crease of your cheeks is ideal,

SEND HIM THE TEASER!

TYPE THE LINK BELOW. CASE SENSITIVE.

101nights.com/ VivaLaJuicy

FOR HER EYES ONLY

NO. 70

ALL MOUTH

101 NIGHTS OF GREAT SEX

It's very porn star-ish because you're going to make over-exaggerated movements. Lift his penis to expose his testicles, then starting at the lowest part on the underside, stick out your tongue so he gets a good look at the action, and give one long, lascivious lick from the base of his testes to the top of his penis.

5. Make Like A Naughty Starfish

Reach between his legs with one hand, while lightly holding his penis with the other and stroke the perineum, letting your fingers naughtily stray around his anus. It's a hot spot for men, even if they are a little scared. (Hot Hint: The male G-spot is about two knuckles deep. I double-dare you!)

6. Go Nuts

Then move onto some ball games. Take one or both testicles in your mouth, hum lightly, suck gently and swirl your tongue around them. Make sure your other hand continues to hold his (by now throbbing!) penis, but not too firm or too practiced.

7. The Cunning Combo

Using one hand, make a loose fist and start to pump his penis, up and over the head, making sure things are nice and slippery (use your own saliva, or even sexier, get him to spit on your fingers). Now, add your mouth—it's the combination of the tease, firm fingers and a soft, warm, oh-so-longed-for mouth which is what makes this feel exquisite.

8. Twist & Flick

Use your hand and mouth simultaneously; starting to twist your fist once it reaches the head and swirling the flat of your tongue around the rim of the head at the same time. Flick his fraenulum (the stringy bit on the underside, between the shaft and head) with a tensed tongue.

9. Be a Boy Scout

When he's *almost* at the point of no return, pull back, fix him with a sultry stare, then make like a boy scout, holding your palms straight, facing either side of his penis and roll and rub them together, as if you're trying to start a fire with sticks.

10. A Corkscrew Climax

Moving onto the Grand Finale: '*The Corkscrew.*' Hold the base of his penis with one hand and take a firm hold of the shaft with the other, hands facing in separate directions. Start at the bottom and slide to the top using a circular-twisting motion as you wind towards the head. Your hands are moving in separate directions—his head is spinning off his shoulders in pure ecstasy!

Follow my instructions, and you're going to give your guy the kind of oral sex he's only dreamed about. He'll be shocked. He'll be in head-job heaven. He'll wonder where you learned to be so deliciously naughty. And best of all, he'll be more than ready to return the favor.

INGREDIENTS

1 hot mouth (yours)

1 willing penis (his)

2 hands

1 wicked expression and attitude

lubricant or saliva

SPECIAL NOTE:
These instructions are a mouthful so highlight and memorize or better yet, make a cheat sheet and stash somewhere for easy viewing. Good luck!

SEND HIM THE TEASER!

TYPE THE LINK BELOW. CASE SENSITIVE.

101nights.com/AllMouth

TRACEY COX IS ONE OF THE MOST PROLIFIC SEX authors in the world. In total she's written 15 books on sex, flirting and being one hot mama. I asked Tracey to provide my readers with her best oral tricks. Here's one Night of Great Sex in Tracey's words:

It's Friday night. He walks through the door after a long week. Hand him a beer, take his laptop, unzip his fly, and then drop to your knees—it's the only *true* position to deliver gobsmackingly great oral sex. Why? First up, you're kneeling before him, worshipping the piece of him he's most in love with and so presumes you are too—his penis. Plus it's terribly politically incorrect and anti-feminist— he tries his best to be the opposite most of the time, but it's nice to let loose his "Me Tarzan, You Jane" primal side once in a while!

Now, before you even think about wrapping that hot, delicious mouth of yours around him, get *your* head around these must-follow tips to give him the best oral sex he's had in his whole life— all in one go!

1. Look Like You Love It!
You need to let him know you love what you're doing. Make faces, grimace, do anything but lick with relish and the whole thing is utterly pointless!

2. Clothes *On* Please!
Make sure you're clothed while he's naked. This adds to the power play—you're on your knees but he's stripped bare, delivering a delicious combination of strength and weakness.

3. Eye Him Off
Make and hold eye contact as much as possible. Most women keep their eyes closed during fellatio, and blatantly eyeing him off while you're being such a hussy is a turn-on for both of you!

4. The Lollipop Lick
Start by playing porn star and doing '*The Lollipop.*'

NO. 71

EVERYTHING & THE KITCHEN SINK

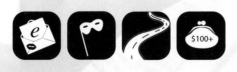

invite him to distract you while you attempt to concentrate on your task. He can have his fun making you lose your concentration, and possibly total physical control.

Of course, you're already prepared a set of kinky playthings to make distracting you more inviting. On the counter next to you—oh, don't worry, he'll notice—you've set out your favorite lubricant or oil, a feather duster, small vibrator, and wooden spoon. Be sure that you're cuffed or tied to the sink loosely enough to wiggle, or get free if he can't make it home at the agreed-on, appointed time. If you lock yourself in with keys, place one within your reach, but tell him your only way out is the key (a duplicate) you've got across the room on the kitchen table. And it seems you can only be set free once you've done your duties.

You're totally at his mercy to be oiled up, smacked on the bum with the spoon for not getting the wine glasses clean enough, tickled with feathers, or buzzed into bliss while you beg to be left to your chores. Or, he may decide you're the dirtiest thing in sight and that you need a good soaping up with that warm water and suds. Before he has his way with you, of course.

Not only will neither of you look at the kitchen the same way again, you won't believe what an unexpected set-up like this can do for your dynamic. It will take you and your man to new heights of playfulness.

When you're through with the dishes, tell him it's his turn to "get clean." With tongue or hands, unless he sets you free, you're at his service.

INGREDIENTS

1 corset or bustier

1 maid's cap, obtained at your local (or online) costume supply store

1 set of cuffs or soft nylon rope (and scissors for quick rope release)

1 bottle of oil or sexual lubricant

1 small battery-powered (preferably waterproof) vibrator

1 feather duster

1 wooden spoon

your highest heels

lots of dirty dishes

plenty of soap

warm kitchen

USUALLY THE ONLY THING YOU FEEL AFTER CLEANING UP the kitchen is relief—that it's over. But in this seduction, getting the dishes done has never felt so good.

You've already let him know that when he comes home, there will be a private surprise waiting for him in the kitchen. He'll likely think you're cooking—a mess that will only have to be cleaned later. But when he walks into the kitchen, there's a scene he'd never imagine—you, wearing nothing but high heels, a corset and a maid's cap, busily washing dishes. Tied to the kitchen sink.

Acknowledge him with a casual "*Oh, hi.*" over your shoulder so he can see that you're indeed his dutiful maid—and sex prisoner. When he walks over to see what you're up to, he'll find that you've carefully cuffed (or tied) yourself to the sink. Tell him you're really just trying to get the house clean, but are trapped doing dishes. Ask if you're getting the pots and pans clean enough. Let him know you're just trying to do a good job, and mind your business while doing your chores. The point is to

SEND HIM THE TEASER!

TYPE THE LINK BELOW. CASE SENSITIVE.

101nights.com/
EverythingAndKitchenSink

NO. 72

JUST A
BREATH AWAY

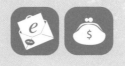

few drops of *Nag Champa* oil; its exotic, peppery scent is *made* for deep inhalations)
- Change the sheets while she's bathing
- Light a few candles in the bedroom
- Burn some incense to create an exotic atmosphere
- Change the lightbulbs to blue
- Put on some mood music (Try Ravi Shankar, Hearts of Space or Enigma-Principles of Lust)

When she's done with her bath, meet her in the bathroom wearing only a towel and wrap her in one as well. Take her hand and lead her into the bedroom, *Honey, let's breathe together for fifteen minutes...* When she sees the scene you've set for her—the candles, the incense, the music playing softly—she won't be able to drop her towel fast enough! Go through the positions in order, staying in each one for 5 minutes.

Position #1: Lean On Me
Lead her to the bed, drop your towels and sit with your back propped against the headboard with some pillows, legs apart. Have her sit between your legs and relax with her back on your chest. Now start synchronizing your breathing. Inhale the smell of her skin and hair as she leans into your chest, feeling your heartbeat.

Position #2: Spoon Me, Baby
Move down so that you're spooning together on the mattress with her body in front of yours, her body still snuggled into your chest. Continue to breathe together, and move your hips in rhythm with your breath. Your erection is pressed against her, and can slide right between her thighs. So close, so tempting, but you're still building up to the main event. Stay five minutes here, keeping your breaths together, gently stroking her shoulders, caressing her breasts and resting your hand over her mound as you move your hips in unison.

Position #3: Love in Legoland
Now you're feeling energized, your Buddha is awake and excited, and you're ready for five minutes of penetration. Sit against the headboard, with pillows behind your back. With your feet on the mattress, legs apart, pull her into your lap, facing you. Put her hands behind your neck and guide your shaft into her. Nice. And deep.

Don't move. Hold your lover in your lap, wrap your arms around each other and take a moment to get used to the feeling. You're stuck together like Legos now; there is no space between your bodies. You're holding her securely, and the feeling of weightlessness she gets is incredible, trust me. Take a few breaths together, face to face.

Then start to slowly rock yourselves back and forth. Your penis rubs against her G-Spot, while your pubic bone gives her clit something to move against; a magical combination when it comes to female orgasms. It may be a new sensation for your penis to be pulled in different directions while inside her—enjoy it—and her response. The deeper your breathing, the easier it is to relax and let your orgasms rush through your bodies, exploding into a million stars above your heads.

Who's up for a yoga class?

NO.72 JUST A BREATH AWAY

INGREDIENTS

candles

incense

a sheer scarf or blue light bulbs

Relaxation sounds on Spotify

"IF YOU EXPERIENCE AN ERECTION LASTING LONGER THAN FOUR HOURS…"

…Call your buddies and tell them how! Seriously, though, what if I told you there are men who *can* last that long, and without any little blue pills? And, no surprise, their partners are *very* happy.

The simple secret to stamina is Tantra. Tantric sex takes years to master, but relax; I'm not sending you to yoga class…yet. This week I'm teaching you a five-minute breathing technique that is virtually guaranteed to give you and your lover the orgasms of the century, no blue pills required.

It's simple: *Breathe in and out through your nose.* Try it now, by yourself. You automatically have to breathe more slowly and controlled, right? You breathe more deeply. Hey, look at that, you're already more relaxed. Keep breathing like that for five minutes. That's it.

That's it? Yes, but it takes two to tango and you'll need a partner. This week you're going to practice that breathing technique in *three sexual positions* with your girl. After fifteen minutes, your neighbors will be wishing for earplugs.

Titillate her each day with quote or a video from one of the many Tantra websites online. Make sure to send her an article on the definition of Tantra, one about breathing (there are several), and one or two different techniques you're interested in. She'll definitely be intrigued, and will take a peek around for herself. Keep it *simple*; this interlude is to give you both a taste of Tantra and whet your appetites for more.

On Friday send her an a text that says: *I've been really getting into this Tantra stuff. What do you say we practice Tantric breathing together? Tomorrow at 9?* She'll be stunned and more than ready for your exotic surprise.

Here's how you get ready:
- Take a shower (women love a clean man)
- Draw her a bath with her favorite bath oil (or try a

SEND HER THE TEASER!

TYPE THE LINK BELOW. CASE SENSITIVE.

101nights.com/
JustABreathAway

NO. 73

THRUST RELAX REPEAT

It turns out that the rule of nines is said to be an ancient Taoist sex trick. The man is not supposed to withdraw but instead maintain a "seal" with his partner at all times. Couples are advised to coordinate their breathing with each stroke; he exhales, she inhales. Alternative methods are three shallow, one deep; six shallow, two deep, etc.; one centimeter, then two, then three, etc.; or simply continuing with nine shallow and one deep until you reach 1,000 (good luck).

This trick is so satisfying for your woman because it makes you slow down, while the shallow thrusts stimulate her clit. You're forced to tease your partner with your erection, and in turn, you're teasing yourself.

This week, introduce the rule of nines to your unsuspecting partner. First, send her the Teaser created especially for this seduction. The teases work like magic. The second she sees it, she starts thinking about sex, which is always a good thing. Set up your sex date and plan on surprising her with a few of your own tricks. This book should be inspiring you to get creative...so get creative! Then when the moment is right, when you're in no rush—because for this to be most effective, you'll need to take your time—start by kissing her slowly and passionately. Have her lie on her back on the bed while you stand next to it; use a pillow under her ass to raise her butt up a little. Also, don't count out loud or move your lips! If she gets suspicious, tell her that you are concentrating on her pleasure tonight, and that she should enjoy herself. She'll wonder what's up, but in due time, the rule of nines will work its magic.

So my new Taoist master… go count your strokes and she'll count her blessings.

NO.73 THRUST RELAX REPEAT

INGREDIENTS

you

her

your left brain
(to keep count)

CHIP ROWE ISN'T JUST THE MOST RENOWNED and respected Playboy Advisor in the publication's history. He's one of the most widely read advice columnists of all time—10 million readers in 14 countries, to be exact. He's helped millions of men (and women) spice up their love life, so when I asked him to contribute one of his best ideas to my best-selling book *101 Sexy Dares*, he didn't hesitate. And, of course, I was thrilled, because when the Playboy Advisor tells you this is one of the "best techniques" Playboy has ever published, you know it's got to be good. Here's what he wrote:

> A woman wrote to the Playboy Advisor asking whether he or the editors at *Playboy Magazine* had heard of this mythical rule, which she described this way:
>
> "During intercourse, a man makes nine shallow thrusts and one deep one, followed by eight shallow and two deep, seven shallow and three deep, etc., until he reaches one shallow and nine deep and begins again. In my experience this is not as methodical as it sounds. The longer shallow sequences get me off, after which my husband starts again with deep thrusts, which get him off."

SEND HER
THE TEASER!

TYPE THE LINK BELOW. CASE SENSITIVE.

101nights.com/
ThrustRelaxRepeat

NO. 74

HOT PURSUIT

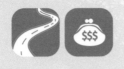

You will need to do a little preparation. Purchase a blank greeting card. Write on the inside of the card:

You have such a beautiful smile. Please kiss the card here, and write your address under your kiss.

Take the card with you to the grocery store at 5PM. When you see her on the aisle, walk near her. Don't acknowledge her. Just read some cards near her. Maybe bump into her accidentally. Brush up against her. After a little while, with the card you wrote, walk up to her, say something like, "I think you will like this card." Give your card to her, and walk away.

She will be beaming with excitement. Her eyes will say it all.

Then immediately go to the flower shop. Purchase a single hot pink rose (which is more unexpected than a classic red rose), and wait for her to show up. Keep the rose at the counter. Walk around the flower shop. Again, brush by her, maybe make a comment to her like "I love the smell of roses." Casually go back to the counter, get your rose, and nonchalantly walk to her and give her the rose.

Did you just hear her gently gasp for breath? Did she just moan? Leave the flower shop.

Arrive at the restaurant bar a little after 6PM. She will be seated with the card and flower. Find a seat across the bar. Smile seductively at her.

Eventually walk around the bar, and ask, *"Is this seat taken?"* Sit next to her.

Compliment her on the flower. Ask how she got it. After a while, ask if the two of you could go back to her place. If she says yes, and she will...ask if she has something with her address on it. Surely she will give you the card with the red lipstick kiss...With your arm around her, and a swagger in your step...Walk her out of the restaurant, and into your passion.

NO.74 HOT PURSUIT

INGREDIENTS

1 red rose

1 local grocery store with a greeting card aisle

1 local flower shop near the grocery store

1 restaurant with a nice bar

1 greeting card with instructions inside

1 good old fashioned email

TIP:
Save this seduction for a special occasion such as an anniversary or Valentines Day.

YOU ARE HER ONE AND ONLY. She is safe in your arms, and she knows it. You give her that security. That's what she has in her relationship with you. Or does she? Sometimes a little mystery is fun to put into the love...let her rediscover you...bit by bit...who knows what new sparks will fly.

Set a date for what will become: A hot pursuit.

On the morning of the seduction send her a good old fashion email, that reads:

> *My love...*
>
> *Today, I'm going to be a total stranger to you, and you to me! Your task is to follow the instructions below. Remember, wherever you see me, don't acknowledge me. We will discover each other for the first time, all over again.*
>
> *1) 5 PM _____ Grocery Store (you add the address here)*
>
> *Be on the greeting card aisle, reading greeting cards. Be sure to be wearing red lipstick.*
>
> *2) 5:30 PM _____ Flower Shop (you add the address here)*
>
> *Browse the flowers—don't arrive early.*
>
> *3) 6 PM _____ Restaurant (you add the address here - pick a nice bar)*
>
> *Have a seat at the bar—order a drink. Be sure you bring anything you have been given today, with you to the bar, and place those things on the bartop in front of you.*

SEND HER THE TEASER!

TYPE THE LINK BELOW. CASE SENSITIVE.

101nights.com/HotPursuit

FOR HER EYES ONLY

NO. 75

CATWALK

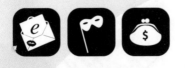

101 NIGHTS OF GREAT SEX

The great thing about this surprise is that you can spring it on him anytime—no set up needed. You might want to save his one for Halloween but why wait? I recommend capturing him just out of the shower. He'll be all warm and clean, and dripping just a little.

Walk into the bathroom in your gorgeous cat suit. Sidle up to him and rub your body against him. Don't be surprised if he doesn't react at first—he's going to be trying to wrap his head around this gorgeous creature in his bathroom coming onto him. He's checking out the boots, how amazing your legs look rising out of them. Your naked ass. The ears in your hair. And you can be sure that he's got his eyes on other little kitty of yours, the one that's just waiting for him to pet it.

Nuzzle his neck and his shoulders. Do like a cat in heat, and press and wiggle your butt against him. He's going to love the way your curves feel. Lick his stomach and chest with long, slow licks. Do the same with his penis—the warmth of your tongue combined with the cool air is an exotic, arousing sensation to men. Watching you half-naked while you give him a blow job is going to be like catnip for him. It won't be long before he's addicted!

When he touches you—and you know he won't be able to help himself—respond with a long, sexy purr so he knows how much you like it. Let him stroke your hair—on your head, between your legs. Use your claws lightly on his back and give him quick little nips all over his body.

Let him lead you into the bedroom for some amazing sex. After all, you've just become his purr-fect plaything—and while you don't have to come when he calls, you just might want to.

INGREDIENTS

1 pair thigh-high or knee-high boots

1 choker necklace with charm or other "collar" type necklace

kitty ears

bra and panties

IS IT ANY WONDER THAT SEXY KITTY COSTUMES are a favorite for Halloween party goers? Or that so many of us harbor fantasies of dressing up as Catwoman in that sexy skintight black suit? Just recently I watched an episode of *The Real Housewives of Beverly Hills* when three of the ladies dressed up in kitty costumes for an over-the-top Halloween party. And it was pretty clear their husbands couldn't have been more turned on. Or think way back to Madonna in one of her prime early-'90s moments: crawling across the floor to lap up some milk in the "Express Yourself" video.

Even the puss-in-boots character in *Shrek 2* was sexy, with his Spanish accent and luscious purr. And kitty cat vocabulary is luscious, erotic and filled with double-entendres. Kitty. Pussy cat. Purr. Claw. Meow. Stroke.

This is your chance to fulfill your feline fantasy—and stoke his every desire while you're at it. For this seduction, you're going to wear just your sexy boots, kitty ears, bra and panties, and a collar-style necklace that shows him that you belong to nobody but him. Catwoman's latex suit is surely sexy, but she's got nothing on you in this outfit.

SEND HIM THE TEASER!

TYPE THE LINK BELOW. CASE SENSITIVE.

101nights.com/Catwalk

NO. 76

OBSTACLE COURSE

When the time comes, meet her at the bedroom door with your own blindfold in hand. Ask her to help tie it around your head. Then blindfold her, too. And then… turn out the lights.

Now you are both completely in the dark. Carefully, very carefully, lead her to the bed (if you can find it without tumbling on top of each other. Not that it would be a bad thing!). Sit down where you can. Giggles turn to uncontrollable moans as you feel your way to her face and kiss her. Tell her you have a treat for her, and all she has to do is open her mouth and trust you. Carefully, very carefully, reach over to the tray table you set up earlier, pick up a morsel, and slide it past her lips. *Yum!* Can she tell you what it is? Pop a different treat into her mouth. What's that one? Put one in your own mouth and transfer it to hers with a kiss. Eat, and kiss, and eat again.

Things start to get trickier now. You've got to undress her by touch. It's not as easy as you think! Unsnap, unzip. Lift and tug. But all those obstacles make the end result that much more rewarding.

Move your kisses to unexplored territory. Nuzzle and lick and find your way around without using your eyes. Feel your way to her breasts. Guide her hands to your penis. Navigate her body by taste and smell. Rediscover the beauty of her hips and her belly. Focus on the scent and the deliciously tangy taste of her sex. Oh, and that sound, that glorious pornographic *slurp* as she takes you deep into her mouth; is there anything as arousing as that? Her hair tickles your thighs with every bob of her head. Tonight, your fantasies fly blind.

You've made love in the dark before, but doing it in utter blackness is different. It's *funnier*, for one thing. It's hotter. And everything about it—including *you*—is a little bit harder.

no. 76 OBSTACLE COURSE

INGREDIENTS

2 blindfolds

tray of goodies

Q: **Why do so many long-term couples have less and less sex?**

A: **Because sex is too easy.**

There's more to it than that, of course. But when two lovers finally get to share the same bed every night, sex is less of a logistical challenge. They risk losing one of the critical components of my famous Erotic Equation:

Anticipation + Obstacles = *Great* Sex

And using the mathematical Property Of Addition, we see that Average Sex can be turned into *Great Sex* simply by…adding obstacles!

This week's obstacle is a pair of blindfolds. Put one blindfold in a place where she can't miss it—the steering wheel of her car or on top of her keyboard. Tape a note to it: *Bring this to the bedroom Friday at 9pm.* Do it early in the week, to give her some time to let that sense of anticipation multiply.

Right before your sex date, you need to prepare the bedroom. Straighten up. Make sure the floor is clear and everything is exactly where it should be. Bring in a tray table of bite-size snacks and put it in a place where you can easily reach it from the bed.

SEND HER THE TEASER!

TYPE THE LINK BELOW. CASE SENSITIVE.

101nights.com/ ObstacleCourse

NO. 77

PANTY DIARIES

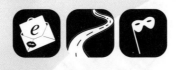

555-2839 LOLA: *I put on those panties u love. Sexy. Leopard print. Wish u could see them now.*

Selfie: *Upclose shot of you wearing panties, maybe with your hand tugging at the side.*

555-2839 LOLA: *Parking lot at work. Thinking of u. I'm a little wet…*

Selfie: *In your car, giving him a peek of your bra or if you've got enough privacy, your bare breasts.*

555-2839 LOLA: *In bathroom at work, wishing u were here, to do me on the counter. Wetter now…*

Selfie: *Photo of your bum from behind, with you looking back at the camera.*

555-2839 LOLA: *Meeting in conference room (sooo boring)*

555-2839 LOLA: *I'm imagining u going down on me under conference table. So hot!*

Selfie: *Close-up of you with those panties pulled down around your upper thighs, touching yourself.*

555-2839 LOLA: *Touched myself under desk at work. Then licked finger like I was turning page, right in front of Jennifer. LOL!*

Selfie: *Pic of you with your finger pressed to your lips as if you're about to seductively suck it.*

555-2839 LOLA: *Need to get ready for tonight. Going home early.*

555-2839 LOLA: *At home now. In the bedroom. Thoughts of u all day make me soooo wet. Can't wait for you to cum and get me!*

Selfie: *Full shot of you stripped down, back to your panties and on the bed, all ready and waiting for him.*

Now take those panties—yes, the ones you have been wearing all day—and wave them through a mist of perfume. Hand them over to your guy the moment he walks through the door. Nod your head knowingly. *"Yes, baby. Those are the ones I was playing in. The ones I wore all day while I was thinking of you."*

Watch his face light up when he realizes what he's holding in his hands. He'll bury his face in them, drawing in their overpowering fragrance (of perfume and sex).

Oh, yes, it *smells just like heaven.* (It smells like something a man would live and fight and die for. Something he will want more of, lots more.) He is definitely going to want to take this shamelessly sexy Lola and make love to her, hard and often, and as soon as possible.

And Lola? She's just wicked enough to let him.

INGREDIENTS

1 vibrator

2 smartphones

your sexiest panties

a little perfume

an orgasm or two

I *LOVE* THOSE SPECIAL "FLIRT-WITH-A-STRANGER" nights when I get to create a whole different character, and then let my guy seduce the new me. I have a couple of wigs I use just for that purpose. For one night I can be a wilder, more adventurous woman, usually named Lola. I'm grinning right now thinking about the naughty things Lola has done.

So this week, find a day when you know he won't be slammed with a deadline or stuck in meetings all day at work. You'll want him to be able to check his phone frequently because you're going to send him a bunch of texts... accompanied by selfies, of course. The sexts will let him know you can't stop thinking about him and the selfies are, well, self-explanatory. No matter how long he's known you or how well he knows what you look like, right down to that sexy little mole no one else sees, he wants to see sultry visuals of you. He likes to know that photo was just taken, in real time, just for him. There's something about the immediacy that makes men go crazy.

If sexting is completely out of character for you, start by explaining how you can't stop thinking about sex since you began doing the book together. Recognize your comfort level. Then maybe push a little past it! Tell him you've been reading a lot of sexy stuff lately and it's making you hot. Start by describing the sexiest day you ever had. And don't just make it up. Live it. Play with yourself all day and share your excitement with him. Something like this:

SEND HIM THE TEASER!

TYPE THE LINK BELOW. CASE SENSITIVE.

101nights.com/
PantyDiaries

Texts from LOLA

555-2839 LOLA: *U just left & I'm still in bed, wishing u were here with me! Guess I'll have to settle for the dolphin vibe!*

Selfie: *Photo of you in bed holding vibe with a sly smile.*

NO. 78

RED LIP DISTRICT

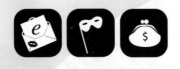

Up close, he sees the rest of your naughty outfit. Under an open robe, you're wearing only panties and a bra. In red, of course. Be bold. Smile as you pat his zipper. Slowly undo his belt. Timeless dominatrix move: fold the belt in half and *crack it*—and watch him jump. Unzip his pants, and let them drop to the floor. Leave his underwear on, and continue to massage the growing shaft hidden inside.

Pull his cotton-clad erection to your mouth and kiss it. Yes, plant a bright lip-print right on his briefs over his twitching penis. Kiss it again and again. Pull it into your mouth and nibble it through the fabric. *Oh. My. God.* Suddenly… *what's that sound?* Yes, he knows! It's a vibrator. You had it hidden between your legs, and now it's buzzing against your clit while he watches you drag your teeth across the taut fabric. After a bit, bring the buzzing toy to your lips and kiss it. Invite him to kiss it, too. *Yum.* Now whisper: *"Bend over the chair."*

Oh, that's *naughty!* Stand up and make him lean forward over the chair. Walk behind him. Compliment him on his lovely *arse.* Run your nails across his bum and don't be afraid to dig in.

Pull his underwear down. *"Ooh, look what I found!"* you squeal, cupping his jewels. Laugh and give them a gentle squeeze. Pull the belt from your robe and tickle his bottom with the silky fabric. Run it between his thighs and tie it loosely around his erection, tugging the ends to make his penis dance and his sack jiggle.

You have his full attention now. The fabric knotted around his shaft, the submissive position, your amazing outfit and strong sexual persona—no wonder the Brits love bedroom games. Even better, this game allows your man to slip into an erotic reverie. He'll do anything you say, not because he's your prisoner, but because it just feels so bloody good!

Give him two more orders. First: tell him to get on his knees, in front of the chair. You're going to sit in it again, but this time it won't be the back of the chair between your legs, but rather, his head. Take your time, enjoy; there's no doubt who's in charge here. You've earned his loving licks. And then, when you're ready: make him lift your ankles high in the air while he slides inside you, pumping, rocking, and making love in the chair until the two of you thoroughly soak the silky belt from your robe, still tied around his tool.

Oh dear. I hope it's machine washable.

NO.78 RED LIP DISTRICT

INGREDIENTS

1 chair

1 slinky robe, with belt or sash

1 red bra with matching knickers

1 pretty hat (fedora, trilby, or beret are ideal)

1 red lipstick

1 pair high heels

3 sheets of paper

1 soft blanket or throw

1 vibrator

1 sassy attitude

SEND HIM THE TEASER!

TYPE THE LINK BELOW. CASE SENSITIVE.

101nights.com/
RedLipDistrict

I *LOVE* THE BRITISH ATTITUDE TOWARDS SEX! Sure, their Queen seems proper and reserved, but her subjects? Wildly open about sex. They joke about it, talk about it, and buy the most fabulous outfits to participate in it. My jaw dropped when reading British statistics on role-playing, spanking, vibrator ownership (highest in the *world!*), and bondage games.

You can't spell F**k without the U.K.!

The Brits are seriously naughty, and this week, you are too. After all, The Red Room of Pain from *Fifty Shades of Grey* was created by E. L. James, another wildly kinky Brit.

To start, apply some luscious red lipstick to your lips and press a perfect print onto three sheets of paper. The first gets folded and left wordless in your honey's laptop. That single kiss will be enough to put a smile on his face and get him thinking about you. The next day, leave another paper kiss where he'll find it, with this sultry note: "I've got plans for you, if you're good. Or if you're bad." Let him find the third kiss Friday morning: "Tonight. Bedroom at 8. No sooner, no later." Your lips will be pressed onto his mind all week.

The moment he walks into the bedroom Friday night and sees you straddling a chair (the back of it facing him), he's thinking: *You look gorgeous. Amazing. Hot.* He can't see your body because there's a luxurious blanket draped over the chair's back and seat, making it quite cushy for you, but blocking his view.

What he *can* see leaves him breathless. The highest of heels, the reddest of lips. You're wearing a hat—which, like all hats, has the power to transform you into another character altogether. In a low, sultry voice, say, *"Come here. Stand in front of me."*

FOR HER EYES ONLY

NO. 79

LOVE RIDE

101 NIGHTS OF GREAT SEX

a steamy song playing low. And to make this image hotter than any car calendar he has ever seen, there's *you*—or rather, the back side of you, framed by the open door. Your feet are on the ground, with spectacular strappy do-me-now shoes. Your top half is fully dressed, but bent forward into the car; you are face down on the driver's seat. And because your ass is thrust high, cheeks spread wide, outlined by the soft glow of the car's interior light, it is easy for him to see that you are wearing nothing below the waist but a sexy little thong.

He may be stunned into silence. This is an extraordinary sight, after all, a man's wet dream come true. Let him watch as your hands slide up between your thighs. The vibrant color of your nails will hypnotize him as your fingers start stroking the tiny strip of fabric between your cheeks, gliding up and down your barely-covered lips, sliding under the sheer fabric to flick your clit. Give him a few highly charged minutes to enjoy watching you get yourself wet, right there in the very spot where he usually spends so much time alone.

Now…invite him to come drive you home.

INGREDIENTS

1 thong

1 car

1 garage (or *not* in the garage, if you dare!)

1 pair of strappy high heels

music

FOR THIS EROTIC ENCOUNTER, YOU'RE GOING TO COMBINE CARS AND SEX.

For a guy, the only way you could make this hotter is if you did it while parked right on the 50-yard line at the Super Bowl.

But I'm going to suggest staging this in your own garage, at night, with the garage light off. That's daring enough. (You daredevils can try to do it with the garage door *open*!)

One evening, when you're about to leave for a movie or a meal, tell him you have a surprise for him. He must wait exactly five minutes, then follow you to the car. The vision he sees when he gets there will scorch his brain:

The driver's side door is open, and the only illumination in the whole garage comes from the dim courtesy light in the ceiling of the car. There's

SEND HIM
THE TEASER!

TYPE THE LINK BELOW. CASE SENSITIVE.

101nights.com/LoveRide

NO. 80

POPPING HER CLUTCH

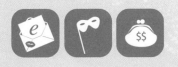

Bring it out in the middle of making love and hand her the egg...but *you* keep hold of the controls. Turn it on slowly to let her get a taste of how it feels. Then turn it off. Uh-huh, that's right. *You're* running the show, and she's gonna know it right away.

Here's a great way to start. It's what sex manuals refer to as the Modified Scissor, and what my friend calls the IncrediblyLazy F**k. It makes kind of an X shape on the bed: You're on your side, and she's on her back at a ninety-degree angle to you, with her legs up and over your hip. It really is lazy; you can rock in and out of her forever in this position. But what makes it great for using the vibe is that her expression and body language are clearly visible, so you know when to drive the controller up—zoom!—and when to back off—gasp!—always keeping her guessing and just inches away from orgasm. Fast, slow, on, off, plus that steady thrust from your rock-hard erection...eee-YOW, that equation makes for hot sex. Way hotter than the vibe alone. See? No competition at all.

For that final drive home, there's nothing more powerful than a trick I call "Popping Her Clutch." To make it work, she has to agree to tell you exactly when she feels her orgasm starting. (Needless to say, the time to discuss this rule is before the vibrator goes on.) Right after, "Oh! I'm coming!"—right at the moment of that first contraction—turn off the vibe. Wait one second, then turn it back on. Repeat. Zap, zap, zap. Do it right and you'll extend her climax far longer than she ever thought possible. Some women report two-minute orgasms with this technique.

And all men report a new-found respect for the coolest power tool they've ever had in their toolbox.

POPPING HER CLUTCH

INGREDIENTS

1 remote-control vibrator with multiple speeds (found in all adult boutiques or online)

batteries

Heads Up!

The remote control vibrator purchased for this seduction can also be used for Position of Submission, Clit Bait, Tongue and Cheek, and Heels on a Dash.

Believe it or not, there are still a few men out there who aren't yet comfortable with the idea of vibrators (we're not talking about *you*, of course). The fear being, I guess, no human can compete with something that never gets tired and delivers the perfect orgasm every time. What I tell these guys is this:

You are completely insane.

No, I don't really say that out loud. What I do say is, *you don't know what you're missing. And you really, really, really should find out. Tonight, if possible. For God's sake, man, your woman is being deprived!*

The thing is—as *you know*, right?—there is no competition. Hey, don't fight the vibrator. Take over the vibrator.

The trick to this week's encounter is the amazing remote-control vibe. There are lots of different models out there, thanks to the ingenuity of brilliant-but-horny engineers around the world. My personal favorite consists of a tiny, buzzing silver egg controlled by a remote or a smartphone.

SEND HER THE TEASER!

TYPE THE LINK BELOW. CASE SENSITIVE.

101nights.com/ PoppingHerClutch

NO. 81

PUSS AND PUTT

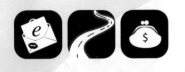

bend *just so*. When you line up a shot, kneel down so that he can catch a glimpse of your well-trimmed grounds.

Tease him all around the course. "What's the matter, big guy? Can't keep your eye on the ball today?"

Just before he swings, goose him between the thighs with your club. "Is that a golf ball in your pocket, or are you just glad to see me?" Yeah, I know, cheesy!

Does this little golf course have obstacles big enough to hide behind? If so, take him around the windmill, out of public view, and hike up your skirt. "Gosh, it feels so breezy out here today!"

Give him a big smile and a discreet pat on his zipper. "You're having a hard time finding the hole today, aren't you?"

Flirt with him. Taunt him. And, if there are no other eyes around, flash him. You're going to have his putter standing at attention in no time. And have I mentioned how many great places there are to take selfies on a putt-putt course? It's perfect for those Instagram photos.

On the drive home, give him a better look at what's under your skirt. Let him see the one hole he hasn't been able to hit all day. Torture him just a little more. Make him keep his eyes on the road while you play with yourself in the front seat.

That's more than enough torment for one man. You've been teasing him all day long. Worse, you *beat him at golf!* So show him some mercy. As soon as you drive into the garage, lean over and unzip his, um, golf bag. Pull out that nine-iron. Give him a lesson like a pro.

Just watch out for that last big shot. It's going to be a wild one. *Fore!*

INGREDIENTS

1 miniature golf course

1 skirt

balls

WHEN WAS THE LAST TIME YOU PLAYED A round of miniature golf? It's been a while, I'll bet. Even in the year 2020, it's still just as fun and silly and easy as you remember, but you will definitely have your sweetheart at a disadvantage when you take him out for a round of Putt-Putt this weekend.

That's because you get to play dirty. And he won't mind a bit.

Right after you rent your equipment, make one last stop in the ladies' room. When you come back, hand your guy his balls. *Wrapped in your panties.* Watch the grin spread across his face as he figures out what's going on.

Yes, you're going *au naturale* under your skirt. You're going to play Commando style. And you're going to win—because there is no way this man is going to be able to focus on his game!

You've practiced in front of a mirror this week, so you know just how to use this skirt to your advantage. You don't really have to show everything. You're a lady, after all, and you're in a public place. Just give him little hints of what's hiding underneath. Place your ball in the tee and

SEND HIM
THE TEASER!

TYPE THE LINK BELOW. CASE SENSITIVE.

101nights.com/
PussAndPutt

NO. 82

BABY GIRL

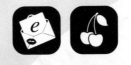

When he's gone, set up a blanket and pillows in the living room. Turn off the lights, light candles around you, and put some sweet and innocently sexy music on your speakers. (You must have speakers, right? Music is so important for a great sex life.) Old-fashioned love songs, like "Let's Stay Together" by Al Green are just as tender as newer romantic songs like "Pyramids" by Frank Ocean..

Put on your most demure lingerie (opt for something white or baby-pink, accented by a bow or some ruffles) and a pair of dainty heels, or even cute white sneakers. Tie your hair in pigtails. Sound silly? He'll love it; besides, you're not going out in public! Put on only a little bit of makeup—mascara and lip gloss will do. Wear just a hint of soft, floral perfume.

Outside the front door, leave a glass of his favorite wine or drink with a note telling him you've missed him. He's going to be expecting something risque, but he's going to be surprised at what he finds: you, lying on the blanket on your belly with your elbows bent, your chin resting on your hands and your feet up in the air.

Sweet? You bet. But sexy too. He's going to want to protect you and do you at the same time. And you can just guess which desire is going to win…

NO. 82 BABY GIRL

INGREDIENTS

pastel or floral lingerie that feels more sweet than sexy

blanket and pillows

candles

music

note

beverage

As women, it feels like we're always trying to live up to an expectation of sexuality: Wear sexy lingerie. Know how to give a great blowjob. Take control of your desires. It's become the mantra for women throughout the centuries.

Taking control of our sexuality can be a lot of fun, but sometimes it's just nice to buck all the sexual expectations and be delightfully innocent. To be free of sexual experience and expectations. To get rid of the sex props and techniques and just be one-hundred percent you. Expose that soft, innocent side of yourself. Think Anastasia Steele when she first met Christian Grey. That kind of innocence goes a long long way.

Give yourself at least half an hour to set up this sexy welcome home. So choose a day when you know he'll be out of the house for a little while.

SEND HIM
THE TEASER!

TYPE THE LINK BELOW. CASE SENSITIVE.

101nights.com/BabyGirl

NO. 83

KITTY POPSICLE

Don't you just love that first rush of excitement as he starts to swell in your mouth? Brush that little devil against your cheeks; swirl your tongue around the rim. Get him completely steamed up, and then—stop.

Is that a look of panic in his eye? It won't be there for long, because now you're going to climb on top of him and slip his penis between your *other* lips. Go slowly. Drop your hips inch-by-lascivious-inch onto his.

Pick up the tempo; let him feel the slap of your seat. But watch his face for *that look…*

Because you're going to stop again. Give him a moment to cool off—and then gobble him up. Nibble and bite and suck, but before he comes, *stop*—and switch again. It's the most exquisite torture. Each time, you're breaking his concentration just enough to slow him down, and each time you're revving him right back up again. Mouth to his cock, which tastes like your vagina and back again; keep it up and in between, let him know how much you love how you taste. Don't be shy. After all, you are the Kitty Popsicle and you taste great. So tell him. When he's in your mouth, make sure you play with yourself, too. Lick your fingers, one by one. Then go back to riding him…and back to oral. Keep it up until the bell rings! And this time, give it all you've got…*Let me have it, baby, I want you to come, I want you to come right now…*

If your guy isn't a dessert person, you can bet he's got a sweet tooth now. Don't be surprised if he asks for seconds.

NO. 83 KITTY POPSICLE

INGREDIENTS

1 kitchen timer (or your cell phone)

1 class in CPR

SWEET PINEAPPLE. BUTTERSCOTCH. WARM apple pie. Peaches and cream. The taste of your pussy can be compared to all kinds of delicious desserts—but the reality? The treasure between your legs is the ultimate treat. You should love your pussy, and the way it tastes, just as much as your man does (and trust me, he loves it more than anything.) Every woman smells and tastes different, and that's a beautiful thing. Even more magical, you have power over your own special flavor. When I want to smell extra-sweet, I drink a lot of fresh juices and eat fruit. It's been proven they, along with yogurt, makes you taste even more delicious than usual.

A few days before this seduction, eat some of your favorite fruits—you'll taste more luscious than ever because you're about to become the Kitty Popsicle! Tonight's playtime starts typically enough, with lots of flirting and kissing. When your clothes are gone…well, mostly gone…sit up and smile. Grab a kitchen timer, crank it to fifteen minutes, and set it aside. Let him lie back as you start to practice your best oral sex tricks. Yum!

SEND HIM THE TEASER!

TYPE THE LINK BELOW. CASE SENSITIVE.

101nights.com/
KittyPopsicle

NO. 84

CLOSE QUARTERS

from her bikini, the freckles along the bridge of her collarbone. She will feel you watching. She will feel your eyes on her.

Right when she starts to tremble, stand and come closer, using only your fingertips to touch her body. Brush her so lightly that she can only barely feel the circles and diamonds you trace over her skin. Make her shiver, but tell her not to drop the quarters.

Keeping her hands above her head isn't going to be easy, but if she drops the quarters, the game is over. Let her know if any fall, there will be repercussions.

Bite her neck. Nip her earlobe. Kiss her at her nape, under her hair. Ask her if she's wet. Make her describe how turned on she is. Warn her not to let the quarters fall.

Touch her everywhere except the split between her legs. Touch her until you can't help yourself. Then get down on your knees and press your lips to her core.

Remind her of the one rule of the game: *She must keep her hands together while you work her.* Make sure she keeps those coins pressed tight between her slippery fingers. Then work her as slowly and carefully as you touched her. While she sighs and presses her hips forward, do not give in. Do not speed up the slow circles of your knowing tongue. Don't let her forget her place. Don't let her forget who's truly in charge here.

Only when she starts to shake, her muscles trembling, do you up the ante. Get one of your fingers wet and sticky and then trace the tip of your finger between the cheeks of her ass, working hard to make her lose.

But if she lets the coins drop, then the game is over and she has to take your place on her knees while you strip off your clothes and put your hand out for the coins.

Win or lose…it doesn't matter.

You'll both come tonight.

NO. 84 CLOSE QUARTERS

INGREDIENTS

5 quarters

PLEASURE ISN'T FREE. It costs patience. It costs willpower. It costs control. It costs a quarter.

Or *five* quarters, if you want to play the game right.

To begin this seduction, call her into the bedroom, and when she enters, start undressing her slowly. Don't tell her your plans.

Have her stand naked, at the foot of your bed. Kiss her cheek. Kiss her lips. Ask her if she trusts you.

Tell her to put out her left palm, face up. Reach into the pocket of your pants and bring out a handful of change. Place a quarter on the ball of each of her fingers, then help her line her right hand on top, fingertip to coin to fingertip. Her hands will be pressed together, with a quarter sandwiched between each of her pinkies, ring fingers, middle fingers, pointers, and thumbs.

Now, have her hold her hands over her head and look up at the ceiling. Really stretch for it. You want her to feel the tension in her limbs, at the back of her arms, and to be aware of the tension that runs smoothly down the wires of her muscles in her back.

Sit on the edge of the bed and admire her naked body—the wispy curls that hide the precious treasure of her pussy from view, the tan lines

SEND HER THE TEASER!

TYPE THE LINK BELOW. CASE SENSITIVE.

101nights.com/
CloseQuarters

NO. 85

KISS OF INTRUSION

Ohmygod. That one little layer of fabric across his lips made this kiss feel different from all the other kisses. It was soft, and the softness of it slid across my lips every time he adjusted for a fresh kiss. The heat of his breath was trapped by the fabric, slowed enough that I became hyper-aware of it—steamy, yummy heat hovering over my mouth, mixing with the warmth of my own lips, cooled only slightly by the red cloth.

I could smell something on the cloth, too, something delicious—oh, yes, he had put a dab of his cologne on it. I wasn't laughing now. I was making out, hard, and I found myself getting lost in the fantasy of it all. Later, I realized what had taken over my imagination. It's something I teach couples about, something I've talked about for years. Among women, the two most powerful, popular fantasies are:

1. Letting the man take charge, and

2. Sex with a stranger.

And here I was, getting surprisingly caught up in both fantasies at the same time. And when I say "caught up", what I really mean is that I was getting completely aroused and quickly heading for my first heart-pounding orgasm of the night.

Not, I am pleased to say, my last.

I've since told lots of women about The Red Bandanna, and they all *loved* it. They got it immediately. Women totally understand the power of scent, the erotic drama of a mask, the sensuous thrill of fabric gliding across skin. They know, each and every one of them, the burning need to just be pinned back and taken by a mysterious man.

So here's your assignment this week. Get a cowboy bandanna, and leave it in a place where your girl is bound to see it and wonder about it. Play with it a few times. Make her laugh. And then one night this week, tie it over your face like a bank robber…and get ready to steal her heart.

NO. 85 KISS OF INTRUSION

INGREDIENTS

1 spritz of cologne, gently applied

1 traditional cowboy-style bandanna.

I LOOKED ALL OVER THE WORLD FOR THE SEXY tricks and tips that inspire the seductions in this book. Except for this one. This seduction is based on a true story that happened right in my own bedroom. It started as a joke, actually; a bit of silliness between Jeff and me. I was in bed after a long day and was, I confess, in no mood for love. Jeff started his cute prank, and—POW. Something amazing happened.

One moment I was giggling and pushing him away, and the next—I was hot. Smoking hot. He did something that shifted my mental image, and I found myself responding to him. The fantasy, the scent, the awesome masculinity of his move--it all worked some magic. And trust me when I tell you that this seduction has the power to take your woman from zero to 60 in three seconds flat.

It all started when Jeff came home after having a cigar with some buddies. I'll never say no to a kiss, but I laughed at this one and mentioned his breath, heavy with the smell of old tobacco. He went off to get ready for bed (and brush his teeth!) and when he came back, he was wearing a Red Bandanna across his face. He looked like a bank robber out of an old Western movie. He had the ends tied behind his head, with a triangle of fabric falling over his nose and mouth. Just a joke. A token effort to keep his cigar-breath from bothering me. But then he kissed me…and oh. My. GOD.

SEND HER THE TEASER!

TYPE THE LINK BELOW. CASE SENSITIVE.

101nights.com/ KissIntrusion

NO. 86

WAKE-UP CALL

Sex Upon Waking. No prep work, no props; the dress code for this party is come as you are, baby. You don't even have to brush your teeth!

After a good night's sleep, you're going to be his personal Wake-Up Call. Set your alarm a little earlier than usual. With some lube, start waking up your kitty. If he hasn't begun to be lulled out of sleep by your alarm, the thought of you rubbing one out right beside him will pretty much guarantee he does. Bring yourself closer and closer to orgasm, while moving your body closer and closer to his. Make this obvious—even exaggerate a bit. You want him to be half-asleep and realize that he's missing out on the hottest thing ever: You, ready for action, and starting without him!

Press against him while you're masturbating, push your ass into his bulge as it grows, lay a hand on his morning wood, and stroke it slowly. Even the groggiest of guys will know exactly what your intentions are, and you didn't have to say a single word.

Then (and he's definitely awake by now, in every sense of the word!), get him spooning behind you. Put him between your thighs and guide him inside. Side-lying sex can be a little tricky, but here's why it's a great wake-up call: You're both facing the same direction, you can keep it nice and slow until you're both ready to blow, and you, sexy thing, are free to grab on to anything: the headboard, his butt, the back of his neck…

Now, I really can't think of a better way to start the day. Can you?

NO. 86 WAKE-UP CALL

INGREDIENTS

Alarm clock

A leisurely morning when you're not rushed

No ONE WILL ARGUE THAT NIGHTTIME ISN'T a great time for having great sex! While getting down and dirty after-dark is so much fun, well, there's something to be said for starting the day off right. I'm talking about first thing in the morning.

Sure, we're more likely to lose our inhibitions post-sunset and well, bedtime can often lead to playtime, but honestly sometimes all I want to do at the end of the day is curl up with my sweetie, watch an episode of *Billions*, and sleep all night. Most women can probably relate. Work and responsibilities take their toll all day, and some nights there's not much left in the tank. My advice on those nights is to kiss your fella goodnight, roll over, and drift off til morning.

You know that hazy, dazed, sumptuously lazy, half-asleep feeling? When you're yawning and stretching and not *quite* ready to wake up? That, my friends, is the *perfect* time to have wake-up sex, also known as morning sex. And I do mean

SEND HIM
THE TEASER!

TYPE THE LINK BELOW. CASE SENSITIVE.

101nights.com/
WakeUpCall

NO. 87

PLAY LIKE GREY

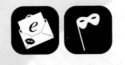

the boxers and bring the rest to the bedroom. Wow! Now he's *really* starting to wonder how much you were kidding. (The answer is still the same.)

When he walks into the bedroom, he'll see a sight that is at once stunning and slightly confusing. Two chairs sit in the middle of the floor, back to back, about three feet apart. Tell your man to hand you the ropes and then drop the pillow at your feet. Make him stand between the chairs. Take one rope and loop it around his wrist, then through the opening on the back of one chair. Tie a knot. Repeat with his other wrist.

He could escape, of course. But he won't. He wants to see where this is going. More than that, he wants to surrender to you. And he won't be sorry he did.

Kneel on the pillow in front of him. Drag your fingernails across the front of his boxers. Feel his package stirring underneath the fabric. Give him a gentle squeeze. Now press your cheek up against the beast hiding inside, and slowly slide your face from side to side. His penis is growing, pressing against the cloth, and when you take the tip of it and place it between your teeth, still wrapped in fabric, you'll feel it twitch. Pull his underwear down, and once his erection is free, slide it into your mouth and work it, in and out, wet and hard. Take your time.

Stand up and turn around. Tease him with your bottom. Rub it against his crotch and then step away. Do it again, a few times. Make him tug on the ropes and shove his hips forward, as he tries to get closer to your body.

Finally, free his wrists and bring him to the centerpiece of your seduction. It's a big mirror, leaning up against a wall or dresser. Put the pillow in front of it and get down on all fours, with your face near the glass. Tell him to get behind you, and *"Put it in me, right now, I need it in me hard."*

And that's when he figures it out. He can have sex with you, and *he can watch himself having sex with you at the same time.* He's just inches away from it, too. It's almost like having sex with another couple, close enough to touch. In fact, you're so close to the mirror you could almost start making out with that other beautiful girl in the room. He loves you, and only you, but for a brief while, he gets to share you with that other guy. He's gone through the looking glass. But this sure isn't Wonderland. It's *wonder-when-we-can-do-this-again* land.

NO. 87 PLAY LIKE GREY

INGREDIENTS

1 large mirror

1 soft rope, 4 feet long
(optional: scarves, neckties,
pantyhose)

2 chairs

1 large throw pillow

candles

optional: 1 copy of *Fifty
Shades of Grey*

COME ON, DON'T DENY IT, I know you've read it (or want to). That titillating trilogy known as *Fifty Shades of Grey*. The series has now sold a massive 150 million copies around the world with the movie franchise crossing the $1 billion mark. But let's ask ourselves why we, our friends, and even our friends' husbands, have fanatically read this fictional phenomenon. I believe there are a couple of reasons why we're so intrigued. One is witnessing a character commit to the act of sexual surrender, giving complete control of their sexual pleasure to someone else. We also enjoy being voyeurs, and reading about a couple's sex life is like peeking around their curtain and watching it unfold before us.

But here's an interesting fact: in real life, the most popular male fantasy is to *be* dominated. So, this week you're going to take on the role of Christian Grey and he's going to live out one of his most powerful fantasies.

Stop by the grocery store and get a short length of soft nylon rope (rope sales have been through the roof thanks to Fifty Shades of Grey). One day this week, hand your guy a knife and ask for his help cutting the rope in two. When he asks what it's for, look him in the eye and tell him the truth. "*Oh, honey, I'm going to tie you up with it this weekend!*" Smile, kiss him on the cheek, and walk away, leaving him to ponder just how much you were kidding. (The correct answer is: not at all.)

Saturday night, tell him you have a few surprises for him, starting with a bath. Once he's in the tub, bring a large pillow to him and put it next to the tub. Place a pair of boxer shorts and the two sections of rope on it, with a note that says *Put on*

SEND HIM
THE TEASER!

TYPE THE LINK BELOW. CASE SENSITIVE.

101nights.com/
PlayLikeGrey

NO. 88

XXXCURSION

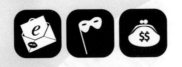

Tell your man you're in the mood to go to the movies and don't worry, you've got the tickets – and the rest! – taken care of. If he protests your choice ("That only got a 69% on Rotten Tomatoes!"), let him know he'll be giving it rave reviews, no matter what.

Now to prepare for your big debut. Before hitting the concession stand for popcorn and Milk Duds, you're going to pick up a special treat of your own: a discreet little egg vibrator you'll be wearing as you slip into the back row. (I told you you're going to turn it up a few notches!) Make sure you wear a skirt for this seduction; the shorter, the better. You also might want to bring an oversized sweater or large wrap to place over your lap for discretion. Now back to that vibrator: Place it in before you leave the house, or in the bathroom at the theater, whichever you feel more comfortable doing. And don't say a word.

By now, you've picked a couple of seats tucked away in the back. The lights have dimmed and the trailers have started rolling. Just like the build-up of a suspenseful film plot, you're going to take your time. Start by acting extra-flirty. Give him a kiss on the cheek. Take his hand in yours. Or rub your hand on his thigh. Let him know you're so excited by his mere presence next to you. Open your bare legs a little bit to get his attention. Squirm around seductively.

Wait until the movie gets going and the theater is pitch-black before you begin your makeout session. If the phrase "tonsil hockey" comes to mind, that's okay! Nothing wrong with a little nostalgia. After things have really heated up and you've unzipped his fly, grazed his growing bulge with your hands, it's time for your plot twist: He's about to realize something else is up.

Reach up under your skirt, slowly pulling out your vibrating egg (the remote control is in your purse). Suddenly, you're the baddest bad girl in school, and he's on the edge of his seat...and the edge of coming. How far are you willing to go? Carefully play with your toy in front of him, as you get wetter. Tell him to taste it, so he can taste you. Rub it over your clit. Trace the outline of his penis with your other hand. You're both so hot and excited now, you can barely keep quiet. Your adrenaline levels are rivaling those of your favorite action hero.

I bet you won't make it to the closing credits. This kind of foreplay is too intense; the anticipation has mounted. By the time you've escaped the theater and made it all the way home, your hands all over each other the whole way, you're absolutely ravenous. Who needs the big screen? Your private show is so much better. You're each other's brand-new crush again—and you're about to give each other award-winning orgasms.

Now that's a theatrical release! And the best part? You've just created a new secret memory to share for years to come: An instant cinematic classic.

NO.88 XXXCURSION

INGREDIENTS

2 movie tickets

1 empty movie theater

1 egg vibrator
(or another type)

some good,
old-fashioned moxie

SEND HIM
THE TEASER!

TYPE THE LINK BELOW. CASE SENSITIVE.

101nights.com/XXXcursion

You're reading this book because you want to get out of your comfort zone, right? You're committed to trying new things and exploring your sexually adventurous side, right? Absolutely right, Laura Corn!

Well, this seduction invites you to go to a place that's always been pretty comfortable for most of us: the movie theater. I know, *I know!* I'm about to challenge you to do something that simultaneously pushes your boundaries and brings you back to your youth. It's bold. It's a stretch. It's designed to get you in touch with the kid at heart (and then unveil a *very* grownup version of her). When's the last time you made out in a movie theater?!

Remember back in high school when you wanted to be alone with your crush? But parents were everywhere and privacy was hard to find. We all have vivid memories of sneaking into the back row at the movies and getting a little handsy with the boy we liked, terrified of getting caught. In retrospect, that element of danger is what made it so memorable.

Maybe you're laughing at the idea of recreating something you did when you were a teenager. Or maybe you're already giggling at the thought, like you *are* a teenager—and that's the hottest part of this seduction! Along with the fact that getting away with it in it a public, yet actually kind of private, place is brazen, taboo, and a timeless turn-on. This time, you're going to turn it up a notch. Well, actually, a few *very hot* notches.

Going to the movies always serves as a nice escape from reality. Today, you're going to create a much more exciting kind of escape. And you're not going to catch any must-see new release. Instead, pick a flick that's been out for weeks, maybe even months, at a second-run theater or an afternoon matinee when the multiplex is essentially empty. Maybe it's a comedy romp, or a classic romance, or even a scary horror one: Whatever feels right.

FOR HER EYES ONLY

NO. 89

UP THE ANTE

101 NIGHTS OF GREAT SEX

You start in your boxers, and you don't have to take anything off if you lose. There's one more rule, but I won't tell you what it is yet. Agreed?"

He's not thinking about that other, unknown rule. Not at all. He's thinking about how good of a poker player he is, and how he's going to be sitting across from you watching you strip. Maybe he's thinking about the way your breasts shake when you take off your bra. Or how he loves the way you peel off your panties. Once he says yes, tell him the last rule: Every time you win, he has to put on one of your pieces of discarded clothing.

Whoa. What? You can see the panic in his eyes already, right? But just wait. He's going to laugh. He's going to say no way. But then you're going to remind him, "Me. Naked. Plus…" as you run your hand along his arm, "You're such a great poker player that you're going to win anyway. And here, I'll take off one piece of clothing just to give you a head start."

It won't be long before you're half undressed—and he's half-dressed. When you run out of clothes (or he's got them all on), make your last bid a sex act using your clothes. Something like, "I'll use my silk panties that you're wearing to give you a hand job," or "I'll let you tie me up with my skirt and shirt."

And this time, you might even let him win…

NO. 89 UP THE ANTE

INGREDIENTS

1 deck of cards

1 challenge

You've probably played strip poker at some point in your life, right? Or at least thought about it. The thrill and fear of getting naked, one piece of clothing at a time. The chance to watch someone else get naked. It's one of those games that persists because it feels slightly dangerous, a bit naughty, and incredibly fun.

For this date, you're going to play strip poker with your man. But it's not going to be like any strip poker game you've ever played before. You're going to get naked—if you lose. And if he loses? Well, he's going to get dressed. Only it's going to be in your clothes. Imagine him, wearing your skirt, trying to find a place to wear your panties.

In seconds, just thinking about the possibility, his eyes will go wide and his penis will get hard. Now is when you lay down the rules. Tell him, "For every hand I lose, I take off one piece of clothing.

NO. 90

BADASS

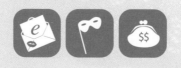

Cover your hand with lubricant, and slide your glistening fingers up and down her warm crevasse. Circle the pink rosebud of her anus. Soon, she'll relax enough for your next surprise. It's not a dildo. No, it's much smaller than that. It's a *butt-plug*— soft, gently ribbed, and no wider than your finger. Lubricate it, and tease her tiny sphincter with it. Press it lightly against her anus, then stop. Work the tip in just a fraction of an inch, then pull back. Play with her bottom; watch how it responds. Take your time spreading her tight hole wider, slipping in and out and then finally…push until the slightly swollen tip of the plug pops in and stays. Leave it alone for a few minutes while she gets used to this wildly unusual sensation. Unless of course, she's already an anal queen, but even then, she's going to love what comes next.

In the meantime, bring out another toy. It's dildo, yes, but not a big scary one (unless, of course, this is nothing new for her and she likes them big). This one is average in size, and once all slicked up will easily slide into her other aroused opening. Gently—move both toys in and out, just an inch at a time. It doesn't take much physical pressure to drive her into a wild fantasy. Tell her to turn over on her back. Order her to hold the butt plug in; command her to spread her legs wide. Now put your mouth between her thighs and triple her pleasure. Move the plug and the dildo, while your tongue flickers across her aching clitoris. Her nerves will be singing, her brain crackling, and in seconds, this ultra-bang will launch her into orgasmic overdrive.

Whew! As one who has been taken there by my own very good bad boy, I recommend going nice and easy at first. There's no need to rush. Whether she's got a virgin bottom (in that case, a little goes a long way!) or an active bottom, every woman loves a man who's in tune with her body.

Like I said at the beginning of this seduction, it *always* pays to be a gentleman.

NO.90 BADASS

INGREDIENTS

1 bottle of lube

1 butt plug

1 medium-sized dildo

IN THE END, IT ALWAYS PAYS TO BE A gentleman. But there's no denying it; for some reason, every woman finds herself attracted to bad boys! There's a dark and deeply erotic side to us that occasionally wants a man to dominate us and make us do wicked things. A bad boy can push our sexual buttons in ways a perfectly polite nice guy can't.

I learned this lesson again recently when my partner, Jeff, found a big bag of adult toys I had purchased while doing research for this book. He's a sweetheart, but something about these naughty gadgets brought out the rogue in him, and one night, he just, well…he took control. I could hear it in his voice and see it in his eyes. I played along, just like *your* honey will, and he took me for the ride of my life. You will have to be bold for this seduction, perhaps bolder than you've ever been. But your lover will respond to your strength and determination.

"Have I ever told you how much I adore your little bum?" After wine and kissing and suitable for play, reach up under her nightie and squeeze her fanny. *"It's true. I love it! In fact, I want to see it right now. Yes, show it to me…"* Put a cushion in front of the sofa, and tell her to kneel and stretch out, bottom in the air. Lift her gown over her hips and gently massage her bare cheeks. If she tries to move, spank her. *"No, I'm not done yet. You stay…"*

SEND HER THE TEASER!

TYPE THE LINK BELOW. CASE SENSITIVE.

101nights.com/Badass

NO. 91

SUPERTEASE

Dim the lights. Put on some music. Disappear into the bathroom and take off your hanging-around-the-house sweatpants and T-shirt. And come back out stark naked.

Have you seen a modern burlesque show? It's amazing. It's beautiful, and choreographed, and it's never as much about stripping it as it is about putting on a performance for your audience. Your reverse striptease should be slow and sultry and elegant. Panties should go up one tug at a time.

Each stocking should be its very own show. Twirl around as you slip into your bra; wink at your guy over your shoulder as you hook the clasps in the back. Shake your hips. Blow him a kiss. Put on high heels and strut around the room. Finally, slide into your tightest skirt, and leave your white blouse open far enough for him to see the bra beneath. And, once you are *fully dressed*…

…make love to your man. Push him down on the bed and unzip his pants. Help him get undressed, and then lift your skirt and climb on top of him. Oh, he has a whole fantasy living in his head by now, something about a powerful businessman and a naughty receptionist who simply cannot resist him. Shimmy on top of him. Wiggle and squirm. Turn around and kneel over his face. Let him see up your skirt. Let him kiss your thighs and your cheeks and your undies. Take him in your mouth. Once you have made him hard, slip his shaft down your open blouse and between your breasts and then squeeze.

Finally, of course, you should straddle his hips and pull him onto your aching wetness, while still dressed. He doesn't need to see you naked, oh no. You have aroused him, and teased him. You have filled his head with sinful thoughts (and a deep admiration for your performance skills). You have put on a show, and now there's only one last thing you have to do before you get off the stage.

And that's get off.

NO. 91 SUPERTEASE

INGREDIENTS

1 garter belt

1 pair of thigh-high
stockings

1 pair of very high heels

1 sexy, office-inspired
outfit

What's the difference between a sexy moment and a smoking-hot, brain-melting, turns-me-on-just-to-think-about-it, unforgettable memory? Sometimes, just a little twist.

Take the striptease, for example. It's timeless, right? Women have been seducing men with artful undressing for as long as there have been clothes. And then, in the middle of the last century, a gorgeous dancer named Lily St. Cyr made a name and a career for herself by standing on stage and *getting dressed*. The act was hot enough to get her hauled into court.

Get ready for your own reverse striptease by pulling out the sexiest items you have, and shopping for new ones as needed. Garter and stockings? Mandatory. Corset or bustier? Sure. And shoes, of course, with heels so high you need a ladder. For the rest, think of Maggie Gyllenhaal's breathtakingly erotic performance as an office girl with a secret in *Secretary*: white blouse, black pencil skirt, wicked smile. If you've never seen the movie rent it on Netflix! It's a classic.

A few hours before your dance, put the pieces of your outfit on the bed. Let your guy see them, but don't explain them at all. When nighttime falls, tell him to sit on the bed and get ready for a surprise.

SEND HIM
THE TEASER!

TYPE THE LINK BELOW. CASE SENSITIVE.

101nights.com/Supertease

NO. 92

BOX OF HOT

Write out your confessions. Obviously they should be bedroom-related and not, *"I ate the last spring roll and blamed it on the dog."* Here are some suggestions. Use them or make up your own; just make them increasingly explicit and risqué as the week goes along:

- I've always wanted to make love to you while you wore white fishnet stockings. What's something I can wear that turns you on?

- I would love it if you talked dirty when we have sex. What are some sexy things you'd like me to say while I'm making love to you?

- I've always fantasized about taking you from behind while you're washing the dishes. Where have you fantasized us having sex besides the bedroom?

- I've always wanted to watch you masturbate. What's something I could do that makes you hot? (Include a toy in the box: something unusual, like a pyrex dildo. They're pretty, inexpensive and easy to clean.)

- I've read that massaging the prostate makes a guy explode during orgasm. I've fantasized about trying that while you give me oral. What have you heard about that you're curious to try?

Again, these are *suggestions*. Place your *true* confessions in the box, one day at a time, and wait for her response.

This week, the atmosphere in your house is going to be *electric*. Starting Sunday, there will be an element of anticipation hanging on everything you say and do. She's going to be on the edge of her seat wondering what you're about to reveal (*Did he just walk to the bedroom? Is he putting something in the box?*). She's going to be checking the box, *you're* going to be checking the box, and *the* box is going to be revealing things that have never been uttered out loud.

On Saturday morning, leave one final note in the box: *I want to make your fantasies come true*. Meet me in the bedroom, 8pm. Saturday night, you're going to fulfill *her* fantasies, and the box has told you exactly how. She's going to be wet all day just thinking about it. Remember, *don't talk about the box*. Don't text her about the box, either. Your personal handwritten notes are what makes this so appealing. Just look at her and share a knowing smirk throughout the day.

Before your date, set the scene using *her confessions* as your guide. Make the bed, dress in something she thinks is sexy, have any toys you might need within arm's reach, light candles.

Don't speak; honestly, there's no need. The box has told you exactly what *her* box wants and now it's time to deliver.

NO. 92 BOX OF HOT

FINISH THIS SENTENCE: A woman will be putty in your hands if you give her _____.

A car? Nope, try again. *Diamonds?* Nice, but not what I'm looking for. No, the answer is *honesty.*

Women value honesty. With honesty, comes trust. And with trust, you can tell each other *anything.* Believe me, that kind of honesty and vulnerability is hot.

Now, here's something to consider: The majority of American women say they wish they knew exactly what their men want sexually. We *want* our men to be more honest about what turns them on.

It's difficult, though, to look your love in the eyes and tell her what you really want. It's much easier to *write* what gets you off than it is to say it out loud. This week, you're going to share your kinky confessions, and you don't have to say a word. And for that, you'll need a box.

A fabric-covered, photo storage box is perfect, but there are endless types of boxes available on Amazon. As long as it's roughly the size of a shoebox and has a lid, you're set. On Sunday, put the box in the middle of your bed. Attach a note on the lid that says, *"Open Me."*

Inside the box is a sheet of paper titled "Fantasy Box Rules." On it, write the following: *This is our Fantasy Box. I want to share my fantasies with you. Every morning I will confess one of my secret fantasies, and ask you a question. You'll have until that evening to answer the question. Here are the rules: 1. We will keep our minds open while reading each other's secrets. 2. We will not talk about the box, and 3. A closed lid means there's something in the box. If you agree to the rules of the Fantasy Box, put it on your dresser with the lid open. I love you.*

Her heart is going to speed up when she realizes what you've organized, and she's going to wish she'd thought of it!

SEND HIM THE TEASER!

TYPE THE LINK BELOW. CASE SENSITIVE.

101nights.com/BoxOfHot

NO. **93**

UP AGAINST
THE WALL

You don't have to say anything. Just approach her from behind and nuzzle her neck. Run your hands down her body. Reach in front and open her pants. Tug them down, and then off. Leave on her panties—for now—and play with her bottom. Slip a hand between her cheeks. Feel the heat. Wrap your fingers around the folds of flesh underneath the fabric, and give her a gentle squeeze.

Now pull your hand away. Wait for a beat. Count one, two, three, then—SMACK! Swat her on the butt. *"That's what happens if you take your hands down without permission."* As long as she obeys, give her more massage, more kisses, more fingerplay through the panties.

Let your hands roam further. Feel her nipples turn to pebbles under her bra. Open her shirt and then slide your hand under her bra. Press your body against her backside; let her feel your hard-on jamming up against her. Pull the panties down, just a little, just enough to let your erection slip between her thighs. Now play with it. Stroke yourself. Women almost never admit it, but they get crazy hot when they watch their guy getting off, and here you are, jacking it right against her, just out of reach. She'll be getting weak at the knees, dying to feel you sliding home.

Finally, it's time to give her permission—no, to *command* her—to drop her hands, to use them on you, to take your hard-on and rub it against her clit, to guide it inside. Tell her to ride it, legs apart, face against the wall, bottom bouncing against your hips. Order her to come. Order her to make *you* come.

And enjoy giving orders while you can. Because we all know who's *really* in command here.

NO. 93 UP AGAINST THE WALL

INGREDIENTS

3 teasing text messages or emails

2 pages of instructions

1 sign, taped to the bedroom wall

SOMETIMES, GETTING A WOMAN TO SUBMIT to lust is simply a matter of saying the right words. And sometimes—like this time—you don't have to say any words at all.

Get your sweetie psyched up for this erotic encounter with a text message early in the day: *Been thinking about you.* Follow it up with another one: *Thinking of things I want to do to you!* Then send one more: *Be ready for anything tonight.*

Get home before her and set the scene. The first thing she'll see is an envelope with her name, taped to the outside door. The note inside says: *Go to the bedroom. Don't say a word. Follow instructions.* The bedroom door has another note: *Close the door behind you. Go to the wall.*

The room is dim, lit only by candles. Taped to the wall, about head high, is a hand-drawn sign that looks like this:

Place hands here

Don't even THINK about moving

SEND HER THE TEASER!

TYPE THE LINK BELOW. CASE SENSITIVE.

101nights.com/
UpAgainstTheWall

NO. 94

BOSS UP

rest of her clothes. Reach under your pillow and pull out your hidden surprise: a soft nylon rope or a pair of soft Velcro cuffs. Tell her to cross her wrists in front, and then loop the rope around them. Not too tight. This isn't about fear or force. It's about permission. She has to allow herself to give in, to be taken, to be used for your pleasure. If you're already a pro in the BDSM arena, then find new restraints, something you've never used and she hasn't seen before. Thanks to *Fifty Shades of Grey*, she's imagined using restraints like these—to her they're like props in a play and will allow her to slip into her fantasy of being the star of her own best-selling book.

Tell her to kneel on the edge of the bed, face down on the sheets. She's going to be in this position for a while, so make sure she's comfortable by piling some pillows underneath her. Tell her how much you like her ass. Tell her to spread her legs wider, so you can see more of it. Give her a little assistance, cop-style; nudge her knees apart to show her you mean business. And if she's slow about it, a light smack will get her attention and warm her cheeks.

Now start to have fun. Cover your hands with lube, and let your slippery fingers roam. Keep telling her how much you love this view, how you think about it all the time, even at work. Go ahead, talk nasty. Keep massaging her with your slick hands, pulling her lips apart, teasing her clit. Slide in a finger. Two fingers. Oh, and this will send her over the top: put your lube-soaked fingers over her G-spot and your thumb against her clitoris, and start to circle both at the same time. Can you feel each one getting harder, swelling up against your fingers? Can you see that beautiful ass bouncing as she rocks her way to an orgasm?

Can you figure out what to do next? I thought you could.

NO. 94 BOSS UP

INGREDIENTS

1 bottle of sex lubricant

3 pillows

1 pair of soft handcuffs or nylon rope

THIS WEEK'S LESSON IS ABOUT THE POWER of restraint.

Not for you. No, you won't be holding anything back. It's your lover who's going to find out that pleasure is at its most intense when she is utterly unable to control it. That means you have to take control. You're The Boss.

And you'll make that clear right up front when you send her this text message: *Your pleasure is in my hands. Meet me in the bedroom tonight and be prepared to lose control.* That's a powerful promise. Instantly, she's more than enticed to see what's going to happen and you will not disappoint.

Be strong. Silent. Unstoppable. As soon as she enters the bedroom, start lifting her shirt off, and then—when her arms are straight up and the shirt has slid past her mouth (but is still covering her eyes like a blindfold)—stop. Kiss her harder. Use one hand to pin her raised arms against the wall, and use your other to unzip her pants. Don't let her move while you run your fingers through that trim little patch under her panties.

Now that you've established that you're running tonight's show, lead her to the bed. Pull off the

SEND HER
THE TEASER!

TYPE THE LINK BELOW. CASE SENSITIVE.

101nights.com/BossUp

NO. 95

KITTY
TRIANGLE

long about your upcoming surprise. And a triangle is at the heart of your new erotic play. Three triangles, actually, which form a diagram of the most sensitive parts of her body, like a map of her erogenous zones. A map you get to follow Saturday night.

Tantric sex isn't slow so much as it is *long*, to give you both time to enjoy each delicious step on the path to orgasm.

LIPS
△
BREASTS
The first triangle for you to focus on is the one formed by her mouth and her nipples.

Less enlightened men than you might just twirl her nipples like radio dials while tongue-wrestling her tonsils, but with your raised Tantric consciousness, you know how to tease with gentle kisses and soft caresses. You know how to play with her breasts before they are bare, and how to undress them as if they were a gift from the goddess Shakti herself. *Take your time.* Visit each tip of the triangle with your lips and fingertips, slowly getting more aggressive as you feel her body warm beneath you.

CLITORIS
△
FEET
The next triangle is formed by her clitoris and her feet.

Ahh, the feet—so sadly neglected by most men, and so in need of loving attention. Rub them. Press your thumbs into her soles and massage her tension away. Squeeze her ankles and the muscles in her calves. Focus on her toes, tugging and rolling and stretching each one. A footrub is an awesome experience, and here's why: those long nerves take a little detour on their way to the brain, passing right through the neighborhood of the clitoris. And when those foot nerves start singing their happy song, well, the clit hears them, and just can't help but join right in.

And it's time for you to join the fun.

BREASTS
▽
CLITORIS
The last triangle is the one that connects the other two, the Love Triangle, from breasts to vagina, from nips to lips, and you get to visit all the angles over and over, turning up the heat every time you complete another circuit.

By now, you've put the better part of an hour into playing with your mate. And she's felt your love and attention, literally from head to toe. True Tantricas would try to stay right there for the rest of the night, balanced on that incredible buzz right before climax. But that's a lesson for another day. Right now, it's your job to bring her over the top, focusing all your attention on her clit, spinning slow circles around it with your tongue, warming it with your breath, trapping it with your lips. Go faster. Get stronger. Pin her to the bed; let her feel your Shiva strength while you pour your energy into her pleasure. Bring her to ecstasy and, like the young Tantra students of four thousand years ago, get ready to drink the nectar of your goddess.

INGREDIENTS

sticky notes

your girl

patience and dedication

EASTERN PHILOSOPHY AND RELIGIONS HAVE a following here in the West, but their growth has been hampered by the fact that they can be hard to explain. *Tantra*, for example, has a history that goes back more than 4,000 years, and these days it's splintered into lots of different styles and interpretations. But I think a whole lot more Americans would dive into Tantra if they understood this one core principle:

The girl's gotta come!

Okay, I might be oversimplifying. But Tantric sex is almost the *opposite* of religions that say sex is not for pleasure. Done right (with techniques that can make it last for hours) Tantric sex is considered a doorway to the divine. Think of that the next time you get down on your knees.

This week you're going to crank up your mate's sexual energy with a recipe that's part Tantra and part Kama Sutra, with a dash of reflexology and a light, sweet coating of Corn. Sex is always more fun when you give your mate some time to think about it in advance, so tease her early in the week with a handful of yellow sticky notes. Put one on her steering wheel, and one on her bathroom mirror. Put one on the fridge, and one on her purse. Everywhere she goes this week, she should find cute little Post-It notes that have one of the following things on them:

Three triangles, like this:

And the words "Bedroom. Saturday. 7pm. Love you!"

A *triangle*? Yes, that's right. A triangle adds to the anticipation, because she'll be wondering all week

NO. **96**

FRIENDS, WITH BENEFITS

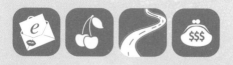

Tease, right?!) The room is glowing with candlelight; there's a pillow on the counter next to the sink. And right in the middle of the pillow sits a single unwrapped chocolate. A special treat, you explain, but she has to eat it without using her hands. And without wearing her pants.

Okay, now she gets it. And she might be nervous about it at first, because there are guests in the house, we have company, *they might hear us!* Make her lean forward over the pillow. Nudge her feet apart. Reach down between her legs; feel the heat rising from her core. Grab a bottle of lube and drip it all over your fingers. Now, use one slippery hand to make yourself hard; she'll be mesmerized as she watches in the mirror. Use the other hand to spread lube over her pussy lips.

Now hurry! Your guests are waiting! Tell her to take that chocolate into her mouth, and at that same moment, slip your shaft into her. *Oh! Yes! Chocolate in one end, cock in the other!* The effect is intense. Breathtaking. And for quickie sex like this, personal lube is magic; you'll be able to drive it deep, and hard.

The sex might be fast. But the afterglow? That will last all the way through dessert. (And you'll think about it every time you see your friends!)

NO. 96 FRIENDS, WITH BENEFITS

INGREDIENTS

1 pillow

1 chocolate

2 unsuspecting dinner
guests

3 candles

personal lubricant

INVITE ANOTHER COUPLE OVER.

Not some distant been-meaning-to-see-you
friends, or friends of friends. No, you want to get
some really good friends over for dinner. The kind
of friends who won't mind if you and your sweetie
excuse yourselves and disappear for ten minutes.
Because this week...you're going to screw around
on them.

Not that they will know what you're up to. But
your sweetie will. The fact that your friends are
right there in the house while she's getting banged
will completely crank up the intensity of the
moment you two are about to share.

Right after dinner, call your girl for some "help"
in the bathroom. She'll know something is up the
moment she walks in. (After all, you sent her the

SEND HER
THE TEASER!

TYPE THE LINK BELOW. CASE SENSITIVE.

101nights.com/
FriendsWithBenefits

FOR **HIS EYES** ONLY

NO. **97**

HEAD
GAMES

101 NIGHTS OF GREAT SEX

exactly, anyway. The object of the game is to come up with clean answers using some very suggested clues. Here's an example:

You read the following to your lover, "*My balls get shot off.*" Huh? There's a clean answer to that? She gives up, so you read the next clue. "*A stiff rod gets me ready.*" Oh, come on! That's got to be dirty. Final clue: "*I sometimes have a man inside me.*" If she's clever, she may figure it out—it's a cannon! And so she gets to draw a card and take a turn.

Now she hits you with a clue: "*All day long it's in and out.*" Hmm, tough one. The more clues you need, the fewer points you get. "*I discharge loads from my shaft.*" Gross! And also no help. "*Both men and women go down on me.*" Get it yet? It's an elevator! And so it goes.

The game is a blast. I giggle myself silly every time I play it. Your sweetie will, too. But at the same time, something else will be happening, something very special. She'll be thinking about sex. The words work their magic, setting up a little telegraph between her brain and her clit. One tickles the other, back and forth, slowly raising her temperature...and her nipples!

Here's another game that will do the same—it's called *Sexual Trivia*, and you advance around the board by answering some pretty wild questions. It covers everything from the obscure, "How many calories in normal ejaculate?" to the surprising, "Which New York Yankee was charged with bigamy?" to the bizarre, "How much does an elephant's penis weigh?"

Of course, word play is only part of foreplay. So kiss while you're playing. Touch while you're laughing. "*Buzz! Wrong answer—time to tweak your nipple!*" After a glass or two of wine and a couple of warm-up rounds, offer to make it a little more interesting. Place a bet. Not for money but for time. Say twenty minutes of whatever the winner wants in bed. Hey, I told you we'd eventually get to the blowjobs! But, even if she beats you, you're going to love losing this game, or my name isn't…

…well, you figure it out: *It's hard to eat me without teeth. A little oil gets me heated up. Pulling my ears gets me off!!*

INGREDIENTS

1 blanket

5 candles

music

snacks and drinks

1 edition of "Dirty Minds: The Game of Naughty Clues" or "Sexual Trivia: A Game of Sexual Awareness" (both available on Amazon)

I'LL BET YOU SAW THAT TITLE AND THOUGHT you were going to get a blowjob!

Well...*maybe*. Hang on, we'll get to that.

No, this seduction is about other games—the kind you need a *good head* to win! I mean word games, specifically, and I include them here in order to make two points. One: For women, words are powerful. Sexual. We can be turned on with the right words. In fact, there are five or six adventures in this book focused on the seductive power of language. And two: Presentation is everything. At least half the success of any seduction is in the set-up.

Who knows why? It's just one of those fundamental differences between the sexes, I guess. It's a bit of a generalization, I know, but women come to bed for the foreplay, and men for... well, for the blowjobs. (Hang *on*, I said! It's on the way.) To put it a little more accurately, everybody loves an orgasm, but everybody goes to it in their own way – and with women, you can't go wrong by starting with *candles and a picnic in bed*.

Make your bedroom look really nice and she'll be knocked out, as much by the effort as the beauty of the scene. Light four or five candles before she arrives for your date. Throw an extra blanket on top of the bed, and set up a tray with a few snacks and a couple of drinks. In the center of it all, place one of my favorite word games. It's called *Dirty Minds* and believe it or not, it's not about sex! Not

SEND HER THE TEASER!

TYPE THE LINK BELOW. CASE SENSITIVE.

101nights.com/
HeadGames

NO. 98

WET & WILD

yourself as you go. Drop the towel at his feet and kneel down to his growing erection. Position yourself so his shaft is directly in line with your mouth. Is he tense with anticipation? Can you feel the coil of excitement in his legs as you grip his thighs with your hands?

Take him in your mouth. Deep, all at once. Feel his entire body growing taut and listen to his intake of breath. Maybe he reaches down and shoves his fingers into your hair or maybe he grips your head with both hands. Let him. Surrender to him even as you dictate the action.

Slide your hands around to grip his ass. Squeeze and knead as your mouth slides back and forth over his rigid shaft. Is he close? Devour him greedily. There's no room for shyness here. Be bold.

Move one of your hands around a grasp the base of his. Penis. Tighten your grip and work back and forth and rhythm with your mouth. Listen to his sounds of appreciation, those primal, male grunts and sighs.

Feel him shutter against you, and feel your power to drive this man beyond reason. Embrace it. Own it.

And when he's finished, slowly rise. Slide up his body, make it flush with yours. Take over his shower. Soap him; clean him. Leave no part of his body untouched. Show him how much you love him and desire him. Then hand him the soap and let him return the favor.

NO. 98 WET & WILD

INGREDIENTS

1 bath towel

A touch of boldness

MEN ARE SIMPLER CREATURES THAN WOMEN. Subtlety is often lost on them. They appreciate bluntness, directness, and an in-your-face approach. So give him what he wants. Be bold and beautiful. Pleasure him…and yourself. Make him crazy with desire. For you. Give him a hot encounter he won't soon forget. A woman who knows what she wants and takes it is a sexy, sexy thing indeed!

The next time he goes to take a shower, put your plan into action. Strip down and walk in after him carrying a towel. How does he look as the water rushes over his flesh? Does he see you right away? Don't give him any time to react.

Run your hands over his body. Wet. Warm. Your fingers glide effortlessly. Let them drift. Take him in your hands, feel him grow hard. Caress, touch, and fondle his balls.

Press your mouth into his chest. Feel the firmness of his skin against your lips. How does he taste? Slowly work your way down his body, lowering

SEND HIM THE TEASER!

TYPE THE LINK BELOW. CASE SENSITIVE.

101nights.com/
WetAndWild

FOR HER EYES ONLY

NO. 99

BOYS
NIGHT IN

101 NIGHTS OF GREAT SEX

Cushions on the floor, pizza on the table, beer on ice. Phones have been turned off. And you — well, you look sexy, but not in that lacy, girly way. No, you're wearing the Guy-World classic: a white t-shirt and cutoff jean shorts. (I'm not making that up. It's the number-one response from more than a thousand interviews I've had with men. They love that look.) Make him comfortable. Feed him. It's okay to let him watch his favorite Netflix show or the game while you eat. Pizza, Pabst, and ESPN…mmm, it's Guy-World bliss!

Slowly turn up the heat. Kiss him after each bite. Climb on him for a nonstop make-out session during the commercials. When you get up for a bathroom break—flash him. Better yet, lift your shirt and press your breasts right into his face just for a few seconds before you leave the room.

Once that first show is over, unveil your special surprise: a mega-hot porno, from a sexy adult website that appeals to both your sensibilities. And as the onscreen action gets wilder, you get bolder. Let him see you roll your nipples through your shirt. Wriggle out of your shorts and play with yourself, legs wide apart, and don't be shy about it—he'll get as big a rush from watching your fingers as watching the screen. Sit sideways to him so that you can keep one bare foot in his lap, gently massaging his erection while he watches the screen.

The rest of your script writes itself. Just follow the action on the screen. Take him in your mouth. Sit on his lap. Stroke him with your hand. Tonight, you are the hottest thing in all of Guy World: His own personal porn star, with an insatiable appetite and a full bottle of lubricant. And tonight, you're going to discover the coolest thing about watching adult videos with your lover: As long as the scenes are hot, he'll be able to go again, and again, and again. And in Girl World, that means you'll be walking funny the next day.

NO. 99 BOYS NIGHT IN

INGREDIENTS

1 sexxxy video

1 hot pizza

1 cold six-pack

1 lucky guy

GUYS LIVE IN A COMPLETELY DIFFERENT WORLD from ours. It's a world where shoes are worn for comfort, not beauty. A place where remote controls are friendly, and tight jars surrender with ease.

Sure, it's a stereotype, but it's one that exists for a reason!

This week your erotic encounter is going to take you to Guy World, and you're going to love it. You'll be creating a little slice of paradise for your man, gathering together all the primal ingredients of typical male life. That's right, I'm talking about the basic elements, the very building blocks of what a guy truly appreciates:

Beer, pizza, and porn.

Whoa! Laura Corn, did you say porn? Why yes, I did, and I said it with a wink and a smile.

First things first: You need to send him a text so he gets a hint of what you've got in store for him. Tell him, "Honey, instead of going out with the boys this Friday night, you're going to have a Boy's Night In with me. Don't worry, all three of your favorite things will be there—and *you know* what they are…"

Even with this heads up, he'll still be shocked when he sees the slice of heaven you've created for him.

SEND HIM THE TEASER!

TYPE THE LINK BELOW. CASE SENSITIVE.

101nights.com/
BoysNightIn

NO.100

LIGHT HER UP

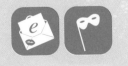

Run the light strands in a big circle all the way around your bed. The tiny white bulbs will make your bedroom look like it has a hundred candles, all focused on your bed like a sort of shrine. Put on some music. Turn the thermostat up by a few degrees (Women are also far more likely to strip down when we are warm). Now break out the massage oil and invite your girl to the bedroom.

When she walks in and sees the glowing lights framing the bed, signaling a spotlight just for her, her jaw's going to drop. Not only will she be turned on, she'll be enchanted. Once she's gained her composure, be explicit: the next hour is all about her. Take your time undressing her. Have her lie down on her stomach, then pour some oil in your hand and get busy.

Work out the kinks in her shoulders and lower back. Squeeze the tension from her feet and calves. Over time, it will become clear that, like all the great artists, you are slowly and subtly moving toward a deeper goal. You're building suspense and approaching your subject from a, um, different angle. After her muscles are relaxed and her nerves are humming, position her on her knees and elbows at the edge of the bed, face down into a pillow, butt high in the air. Now you can finally begin work on her most tender parts...*from behind.*

But don't go straight for the clit. Oh, no. The great artists are never obvious. Instead, tease her by drawing your tongue along her vaginal lips. Up and down. Down and up. Gently suck her labia and roll them around in your mouth. Kiss the back of her thighs. And then bring out your dramatic surprise: *a small vibrator.* This is your big plot twist, where the music builds and changes key. This is what makes your audience gasp. Again, steer around her clitoris. Buzz her lips instead, and her perineum, and her cheeks. Lick some more, then buzz some more. Lick, buzz, lick, buzz—lickbuzzlickbuzzlickbuzz—faster and stronger, creating tension but not letting her get to the point of sweet release. Not quite yet.

No, this story has to introduce one more character before it can build to a climax: *The good guy who saves the day.* He's strong but silent. He's hard as rock, and single-minded. He *lives* for action sequences like this. And he's ready to plunge right in and make everything better in…

The End.

No. 100 LIGHT HER UP

INGREDIENTS

2 strands of small white Christmas lights

massage oil (warmed to body temperature)

hot music

vibrator

HEAD's UP!
The vibrator in this seduction can also be used for Tongue and Cheek, Clit Bait, Position of Submission, She's Out of Control, Lazy Boy, Busy Girl, and Popping Her Clutch.

THE GREATEST WORKS OF ART TAKE TIME to work their magic. The world's most famous films, music and books tend to draw you in slowly, unveiling themselves bit by bit. A lot of times, it's what is *not* revealed that makes great art so interesting. The artist knows that he can create a bigger impact if he makes you wait for the payoff.

Well, this week *you* are going to be the artist. Do as I say and I'll turn you into the Beethoven of the bedroom. The Picasso of the penis. The Hitchcock of the, um, well, you know what I mean. And the surprising thing is that this masterpiece of lovemaking starts with two strands of Christmas lights. Yeah, that's right; Christmas lights are going to help you get some action this week.

I'll bet I'm not the first person to tell you that Christmas lights are romantic. But let me be the first to explain why. It's because women know that we look *amazing* surrounded by that soft, diffused light. And when we think we look good, we are far more likely to get naked.

You've probably noticed as you've gone through the book that great foreplay starts long before you actually start getting it on; it begins as soon as you send her the Teaser. Then on the night of the surprise, make sure she knows to stay out of the bedroom (you can tell her via text or in person). This accomplishes two things: One, it will get her excited! Two, it will get her wet. Telling a woman she has to stay out of the bedroom is like catnip to her. We all want what we can't have!

SEND HER THE TEASER!

TYPE THE LINK BELOW. CASE SENSITIVE.

101nights.com/LightHerUp

FOR BOTH OF YOU

NO. 101

GRADUATION DAY

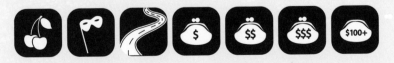

101 NIGHTS OF GREAT SEX

monotony!

Step it up with props and accessories. Fancy or simple, expensive or handmade, it doesn't matter. When seducing your lover, a creative touch says, *I think you're worth some extra effort.* It says, *I don't take you for granted.*

Be daring. Prove to your partner—and to yourself—that there's more inside you than either of you even knew.

All this knowledge is now part of you. And I want you to exercise it all this weekend with this one final challenge.

THE ULTIMATE SEDUCTION:

This one is too big for one evening, or even a whole day. You're going to push your boundaries for the *entire weekend.* And to do that, you need to split it right down the middle. Go ahead, take your pick—one of you gets Saturday, and the other gets Sunday. And on your day, you are going to create The Ultimate Seduction for your partner.

It's going to be easy, because you each have fifty Seductions to inspire you. Start by choosing your favorite from the book. Then add *three extra ingredients* to spice it up. You can borrow ingredients you've used before. (Did you love that bare-bottom apron from Shake and Bake? Do you still get a thrill when you think about the wooden hanger in She's Out of Control? When you think of *that mirror*—or lipstick, or toys, or nylon rope—do you smile? Do you get aroused?)

You can create new ingredients, if you prefer, or make new twists on previous Seductions. Because you know how. You're the experts now. A hundred erotic encounters later, you know *exactly* what turns your partner on. You know which scenario sent her over the moon. You know the outfits he likes to see. You know how to make her feel desirable. You know to make him forget everything in the universe except you.

Your favorite, plus three. That's your assignment. Recreate your favorite seduction, with three new ingredients. Just remember to clear your calendar this weekend. You're going to need plenty of time to play. (And plenty of time to recover!)

INGREDIENTS

Anticipation
Massage Oil
Shoebox
Nylon rope
Smartphones
Texts
Facetime
Leather
Pizza
Lingerie
Bandanna
Tea
Honey
Technique
Apron
Jewelry
Shampoo
String
Platters
Towels
Cologne
Music
Vibrators
Candles
Golf Balls
Showers
Chairs
Christmas Lights
Gloves
Socks
Photos
Instagram
Notes
Blindfolds
Toys
Restraints
Wooden Hangers
Restaurants
Cars
Teasers

and anything else you can think of — you're the experts now!

I HOPE YOU'VE TORN THIS BOOK TO SHREDS. I hope it's nothing but a tattered shell now.

That's because every ripped perforation represents a moment of passion in your lives. Every crumpled page that's *not* here anymore stands for an episode of incredible sex. The emptier it is, the happier you should be.

Can the two of you even *remember* all one-hundred seductions?! I dare you to try. That would be one interesting—and slightly dirty—conversation, wouldn't it? That's the kind of sweet talk that quickly turns into foreplay.

(In fact, a bunch of readers have told me they keep the used pages from my books. What a wicked scrapbook you could make from it! And what a great way to spark up a bedroom fire: Read, reminisce, romance.)

So after a hundred hot encounters, you've had lots of fun, and learned some new tricks. But more importantly, you've developed some powerful new *relationship habits*. By now, it's become second nature for you to:

Create anticipation. You've seen how a simple tease can grab your partner's attention and focus it on you. You know firsthand how much better life is when you can stop constantly thinking about responsibilities, and spend a few moments daydreaming about what your partner has in store for you.

Show surprises. The perfect antidote for

For Catalogs including many of the products mentioned in this book, contact the following companies:

SPECIALTY SHOPS
ADULT TOYS, VIDEOS, BOOKS, SEXY LINGERIE, MASSAGE OIL, ETC.

www.lauracorn.com
(for updates on Teases and Toys)

www.unboundbabes.com

www.omgyes.com

www.amazon.com

www.deepmemories.com

www.a-womans-touch.com
1-888-621-8880

www.venuspleasures.com
1-866-697-5327

www.thepleasurechest.com
1-800-753-4536

www.edenfantasys.com
1-888-506-5516

SPECIALTY SHOPS
SEXY WARDROBE AND LINGERIE

www.jessiesteele.com

www.agentprovocateur.com

www.laperla.com

www.victoriasecret.com

www.lovehoney.co.uk

MORE GREAT WEBSITES

www.parfumsraffy.com

www.marygreen.com

www.jimmyjane.com

www.skatersocks.com

www.spankties.com

FOLLOW LAURA CORN

 facebook.com/Lauracorn101

 @LauraCorn101

 instagram.com/authorlauracorn

WWW.LAURACORN.COM

WWW.101NIGHTS.COM

LAURA CORN BOOKS AND PRODUCTS

101 Nights of Grrreat Sex

101 Nights of Grrreat Romance

You Still Give Me Butterflies

101 Sexy Dares

52 Invitations to Great Sex

101 Great Quickies

The Great American Sex Diet

237 Intimate Questions Every Woman Should Ask A Man

101 Nights of Great Sex...The Game!

The Incredible G-Spot Video